COMFORTABLE, EFFICIENT, SMART

# BACKPACKING
# THE LIGHT WAY

RICHARD A. LIGHT

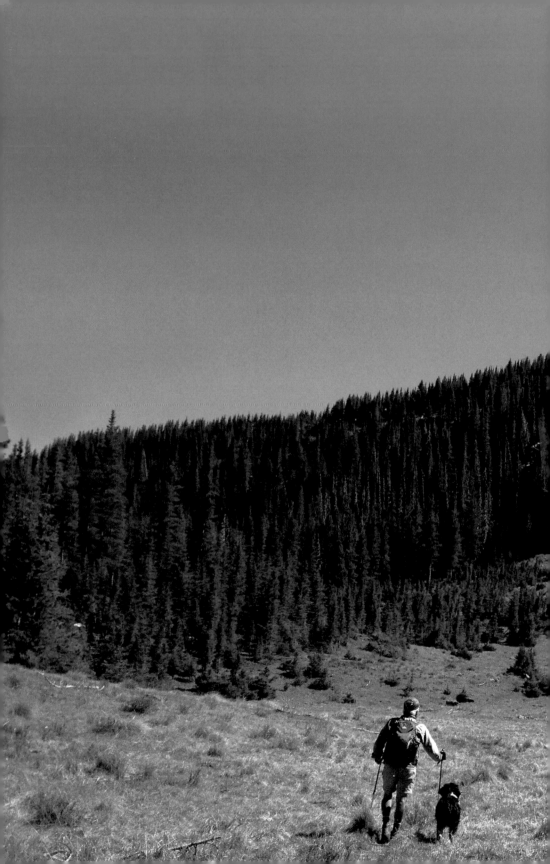

COMFORTABLE, EFFICIENT, SMART

# BACKPACKING
## THE LIGHT WAY

RICHARD A. LIGHT

MENASHA RIDGE PRESS
Your Guide to the Outdoors Since 1982

**Backpacking the Light Way: Comfortable, Efficient, Smart**

First edition, first printing

Copyright © 2015 by Richard A. Light

Editor: Lisa C. Bailey
Project editor: Ritchey Halphen
Cover and title-page photos: Copyright © 2015 by Richard Moeller
Interior photos: Copyright © 2015; see pages 149 and 150 for full image credits
Cover design: Scott McGrew
Text design: Annie Long; original concept by Janice St. Marie
Proofreader: Rebecca Henderson
Indexer: Sylvia Coates

Library of Congress Cataloging-in-Publication Data

Light, Richard A.
  Backpacking the light way: comfortable, efficient, smart / Richard A. Light, with
photographs by Ash Campbell, Thea Rose Light, and Richard Moeller. — First edition.
     pages cm
  "Distributed by Publishers Group West"—t.p. verso.
  Includes webography.
  Includes index.
  ISBN 978-1-63404-028-0 — ISBN 1-63404-028-7 — ISBN 978-1-63404-029-7 (eISBN)
  1. Backpacking—Handbooks, manuals, etc. 2. Backpacking—Equipment and supplies—
Handbooks, manuals, etc. I. Title.
  GV199.62.L54 2015
  796.51—dc23
                                    2015020281

Manufactured in the United States of America

Distributed by Publishers Group West

 **MENASHA RIDGE PRESS**
An imprint of Keen Communications, LLC
2204 First Ave. S., Suite 102
Birmingham, AL 35233
800-443-7227, fax 205-326-1012

Visit **menasharidge.com** for a complete listing of our books and for ordering information. Contact us at our website, at **facebook.com/menasharidge,** or at **twitter.com/menasharidge** with questions or comments. To find out more about who we are and what we're doing, visit our blog, **trekalong.com.**

**DISCLAIMER** Outdoor activities can be inherently dangerous. Neither Menasha Ridge Press nor Richard A. Light assumes liability for accidents or injuries that may result from participation in the activities described in this book. All participants in such activities must assume responsibility for their own actions, health, and safety.

*Walk away quietly in any direction and taste the freedom of the mountaineer. Camp out among the grasses and gentians of glacial meadows, in craggy garden nooks full of nature's darlings. Climb the mountains and get their good tidings, Nature's peace will flow into you as sunshine flows into trees. The winds will blow their own freshness into you and the storms their energy, while cares will drop off like autumn leaves.*

—JOHN MUIR

# Contents

# Dedication

THIS BOOK IS DEDICATED to two extraordinary people, Mason and Betty Light, who taught me through kindness how to appreciate and be fully present within the magic and grandeur of wilderness. It is with humble gratitude that I write in the hope that this work will help others to joyfully engage the backcountry.

# Acknowledgments

NO WORK IS CREATED in a vacuum. With humility, I acknowledge and thank those who have been my teachers and guides as I awakened to the beauty and wonder that backpacking enables. A few of these stand out as major contributors: Bill Kerr and my father, Mason Light, both of blessed memory, who introduced me to wilderness and feeling safe in the wild. Ash Campbell, Rick Kelley, Dick Moeller, Herman Ramsey, and Dave Scudder get gold awards for enduring many years of bad puns and serious backcountry treks together. I learned a great deal from each of them. My wife, Morgan Light, deserves special gratitude for understanding my need to be in the mountains and canyons, and for putting up with my closet full of gear and my many experiments with equipment and menus. And lastly, the management of REI Santa Fe gets kudos for allowing me to create my own courses, through which I have learned more than I expected and have been able to hone my understanding of gear, skills, and people.

# What This Book Is Not

THIS BOOK IS NOT another backpacking gear comparison book. There are many good ones in existence, and gear advances in technology mean today's choices will be eclipsed by newer models very soon. Instead, this book is about navigating the transition from conventional backpacking toward ultralight backpacking. That means the information provided here concentrates on how to make the transition, how to rethink what you now own, use, understand, and expect. This book helps you do that no matter what new gear comes along. It's a complete paradigm shift, yet, with some focus, quite attainable.

Guides, instructors, and trip leaders can benefit from this book, because it teaches proven methods for gear management, effective packing, risk assessment, trek organization, and contingency planning, in addition to the concepts above.

New backpackers and those coming back to the sport will be spared the hassle of learning conventional methods only to have to relearn ultralight approaches later.

The bottom line is that this book will help you have more fun in the wilderness. It will help you carry less on your back while still preserving comfort and safety. Logical gear organizational methodology, along with effective trip planning and risk assessment, make trips more fun. This book is designed to be truly useful.

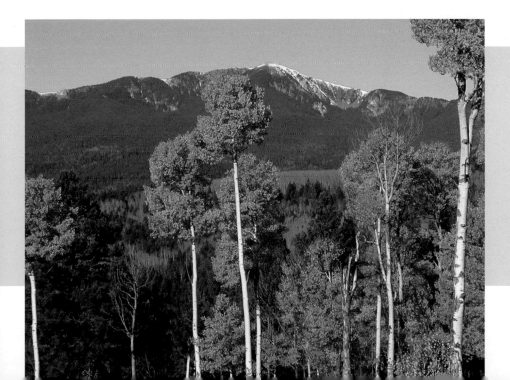

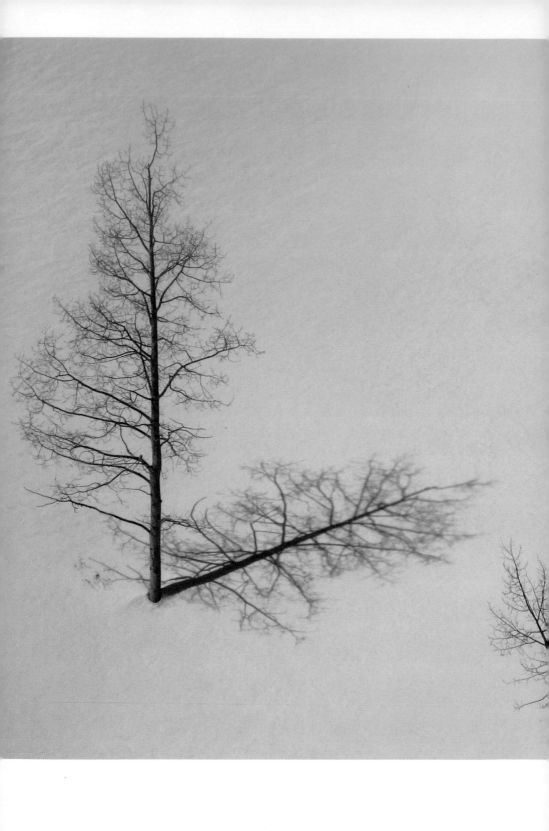

# What Was I Thinking?

IN MY YOUNGER DAYS, carrying 86 pounds was awesome, especially since there were climbing ropes hanging off the top of the pack. They were really manly, and meant that I must be very cool indeed to have them on my pack. It never dawned on me at the ripe old age of 18 that carrying more than 70% of one's body weight on your back might be detrimental to your health. Who thinks of that at 18?

Of course the external-frame pack I carried was amazing, too. It was large and green and had four side pockets and one big back pocket, and the frame was glistening aluminum. The latest, greatest pack money could buy! Or, at least, that I could afford. I bought it through a catalog from a company called Recreation Equipment Inc., in Seattle. The year was 1967. I was in Colorado, so the only way I could touch and fondle the goods was to order them by mail and wait for the magic package to arrive. I ordered a new sleeping bag along with the pack. I was preparing to spend the following summer creating a new company: a backpacking guide service to take teenage kids out into the Indian Peaks region of Colorado backcountry for 10-day treks.

George, a friend of our family who had worked as an Outward Bound instructor, was the director of the company. I was his assistant. We called it Bivouac Mountaineering. We were based out of Boulder, Colorado, and George got the local YMCA to schedule our treks. Over the course of three summers, we took out a dozen groups of kids. Some trips were girls only. For those, we had a third instructor, a woman, who took care of any female issues that came up.

The course curriculum included walking, breathing, how to pack a pack, carrying a pack, how to bake bread over an open fire, cooking over a fire, rock climbing and rappelling, self-arrest on a snowfield, and climbing 12,000-foot peaks. These courses were designed to teach kids about themselves rather than just outdoor skills. We even had them belay each other on a cliff, which was often an awakening experience, especially when the kid in charge of their life—the one doing the belaying—was the one they never trusted.

On one particular trip, I was leading a group of eight boys, two cooking groups of four. Right away, we could tell there was potential for problems. Danny, age 12, was the youngest boy we had along. He came from a sheltered background and hadn't the slightest inkling of common sense, let alone the skills to navigate in the backcountry. Rolf, on the other hand, was a savvy 15-year-old "Mr. Cool" who was not too happy to have to put up with the very uncool wimp of the group. Of course, Danny and Rolf were in the same cooking group. When it was Danny's turn to cook dinner, he took a can of food and simply put it into a pan and onto the fire, without even opening the can. This lack of common skills caused Rolf to react, and he began to belittle and badger Danny, eventually shoving him around until Danny was in tears.

After the immediate handling of this dinner event, George and I separated these two for the evening. Rolf went off to be alone. That day we had climbed our first mountain of the trip: an 11,000-foot peak that was very fulfilling for the kids as an accomplishment. Rolf had been on a high from the climb and then tumbled into a low because of Danny. An hour later he came back from his walk still upset.

I took him aside to sit next to my fire. I asked him if he liked climbing the peak, to which he enthusiastically responded. So I then asked if he wanted to climb a really difficult peak. Of course this got him very excited. He asked, "When can we start?"

I explained that the name of the peak was "Danny," and that what Danny needed was a mentor. I asked if he would become Danny's teacher, guide, and helper for the remainder of the trip. Rolf sat silently in astonishment for some minutes. Then he asked if he could think it over.

The next day, Rolf came up to me with his head hung as if he were in pain. He looked up at me, straightened up, and with a smile said he accepted my challenge. The rest of the trip was a breeze! I'll never forget the transformation in both of those kids over the next week. It was miraculous.

That transformation got me excited about teaching backpacking. And it made me almost forget the 86 pounds I was carrying. But my neck did not forget. I herniated two discs in my neck as a result of that weight. So I am particularly aware of weight issues in backpacking.

Things have changed a lot since then. Technology, methodology, ecology, every *-ology* I know of has grown and developed by several orders of magnitude since the 1960s. Today, we no longer use external-frame packs unless we're carrying wood, or a hunter might use them carrying out some game. Internal-frame packs have become ubiquitous, and for good reason. They fit better, transfer the weight to the bones of the legs better, move with the body, and are easier to pack, load, and adjust. And, they come in several flavors: light harness packs for one to three nights out, heavier harness packs for weeklong or longer treks, and expedition packs. In recent years, a fourth category of equipment has emerged that most conventional backpackers may have heard of but generally ignored as cultish. These are the so-called ultralight packs. (In this book, I use the term *conventional* in relation to the term *ultralight* as a way to distinguish between the traditional approach to backpacking and its associated gear, and the newer, more recent approach that has developed for thru-hikers, or those who hike literally thousands of miles and take minimal weight and gear.)

When I teach backpacking classes, I note these categories of packs and tell people to choose the style that fits how they will use the pack. Mostly, I'm teaching conventional methods to conventional thinking backpackers or new initiates. Ultralight packs and approaches are not included since most folks are not willing to put in the effort required, and because the equipment at our store (I work at REI) is mostly conventional. Yet the desire to make loads as light as possible is always included within the paradigm of conventional gear.

Of course, wanting less weight is not new. I've been lightening up for some years, each year getting something lighter than its predecessor, so my overall pack weight has been going down nicely. But I've been looking through the lens of conventional thinking. I thought I was doing pretty well, having my base weight down to 27 pounds. (Actually my base weight is 24 pounds since I always take my chair and winter layers, normally not included in this measurement.) Base weight is defined as the weight of everything you need except for food, water, and fuel. It includes the pack, sleeping bag, tent, stove, pots, water filter, first-aid kit, and clothing: everything that is not consumed.

I was at the store one day helping a man find something. We started up a conversation. He mentioned that his base weight was 8.5 pounds and he wanted to lighten it up. After my jaw dropped to the floor, I closed my gaping mouth and asked if he really meant 8.5 pounds.

Yes indeed, he commented, and he had all the comforts of home. He was in his 70s and was not about to backpack without comfort. I was intrigued. More than intrigued, I was envious—24 pounds versus 8.5 pounds!

My process of conversion to ultralight backpacking gear had begun. I hope you benefit from what I have learned, and have much more fun backpacking trips.

*—Richard A. Light*
*Santa Fe, New Mexico*
*February 1, 2015*

*A little misery, at times, makes one appreciate happiness more.*

—L. Frank Baum

# Understanding Comfort and Misery

I HAVE BEEN MISERABLE on many a backpacking trip. So comfort and light-weight are something I really appreciate! Ultralight gear and comfort are often considered an oxymoronic pair, yet there are many ways to accomplish comfort. My goal in this book is to help people transition from conventional (and usually heavier) backpacking gear, methods of using that gear, and ways of thinking, to a lighter-weight approach. This lighter approach is based on ultralight backpacking methods, gear, and thinking, but is tempered by (1) the often unrecognized effort required to transition from one paradigm to another, and (2) the desire to promote comfort to maximize happiness and minimize frustration in the backcountry.

All of us have limitations to our physical fitness, our endurance, our strength of joints, and our suppleness. When we exceed these limitations, we enter into the world of pain, possible injury, suffering, and misery. When planning for backpacking, these limitations must be considered in order to ensure our own health and safety, but also to make the backpacking fun and pain free. When I say pain, I don't mean the "normal" pain of being tired after hiking 10 miles and feeling a bit stiff and achy. The pain and misery I'm referring to is that associated with overexertion, extending beyond our abilities such that we either injure our bodies or strain the system to the point of early fatigue, the unpleasant pain of pre-injury activities on the verge of damage. All of us have a threshold at which this pain begins. It's the point at which our bodies begin telling us to stop. If we pay attention to this message, we can prevent injuries, misery, and pain.

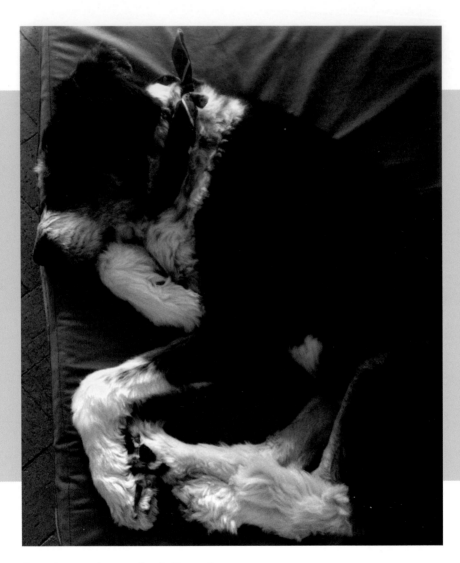

Bruce knows what comfort is. Do you?

This paying attention to our pain threshold could be called finding the "misery index," the measurement of our abilities to carry a pack comfortably on a specific trek. We all have this index. Perhaps we've never known about it or used it, but it's always been there, warning us, guiding us.

Those who have hiked with a full pack know that on some trips the weight of the pack and its effects on our bodies can cause us to reach our threshold of misery: pain begins; old injuries act up; fatigue sets in more quickly than expected. Life is just not fun. This phenomenon is what I call the "misery point" for that pack, on that hike, for the particular hiker involved. The misery point is specific for these sets of circumstances. The same hike with the same pack (or perhaps a lighter pack) filled to less weight can cause no pain, and the hike is fun since the misery point is not exceeded.

My friend Dick, who has been hiking and backpacking with full packs for more than 60 years, relates that if he plans to hike 5 miles with 1,000 feet of elevation gain, then his misery point dictates he cannot carry more than 30 pounds. What he means is that his body and fitness, at his age, allows him to carry up to 30 pounds before it begins to hurt. If he carries more than 30 pounds, he might cause injury to himself. It also means that his experience of carrying the pack is fun for less than 30 pounds, but turns to pain and misery when the pack weight is more than 30 pounds for him on this specific hike.

Dick also notes that the same hike is miserable for his wife when she carries more than 20 pounds. Her misery point is different from Dick's.

This book is about how to lighten our packs so we can stay misery free. It provides the means to minimize our pack weight for specific trips so we never encounter the misery point. By being aware that the misery index exists, we can be more aware on our backpacking trips, noticing when we hit the misery point and taking action to lighten our load so the trip (and future trips) can be less painful and more fun. This book shows how to navigate the paradigm shift in mindset required to create a lighter load. It is about learning how to apply your various misery indices, that is, how much weight you can safely carry under different circumstances. It's a skill appropriate for all backpackers who wish to stay comfortable and misery-free.

*Comfort* is a relative term, and it can be applied to all kinds of backpacking. Let's consider comfort in the larger sense, what comfortable backpacking means. Some people think comfort is defined by sleeping on the ground with a tiny pad; for others, it is only found in five-star hotels. So to be clear, I'm writing this guide from the perspective of a serious backcountry explorer, backpacker, canyoneer, high-altitude outdoor enthusiast, hiker, rock climber, and telemark skier, who, as he gets older, appreciates less and less discomfort in the wilderness. Comfort, to me, means that:

- I don't have to deal with gear problems, and I have more cush where it counts.

- Carrying the pack is a joy, not constant pain and frustration, and it is easy to pack and use.

- I can easily seek shelter from the weather in my tent. I can sit up in it to change clothes, and it provides complete shelter from rain, snow, wind, and bugs. It is large enough to hold both my gear and me, and it is quick and easy to set up and take down.

- I'm warm enough in cold temps (the right clothes and sleeping bag) and have enough padding and insulation underneath me in my sleeping system that I sleep well.

- I have a chair to use rather than leaning against rocks or trees for meditation and relaxing in camp.

- Creating meals is simple, lacks frustrating chores like having to rebuild a stove, and is always reliable.

- Using my gear is fun and supportive of my overall enjoyment of the exquisite wilderness around me.

The above list means I must choose my gear very carefully to make sure it is of high enough quality to meet my demands, is as light as possible within these constraints, and that it fits me well. It also means that I choose to carry a little more than the absolute minimum to support my comfort needs while still remaining light enough to avoid exceeding my misery point.

Because your definition of comfort may differ from mine, your choices may differ from mine, dictated by your needs. As we get further into this, I will discuss how to approach such choices and achieve the comfort you desire.

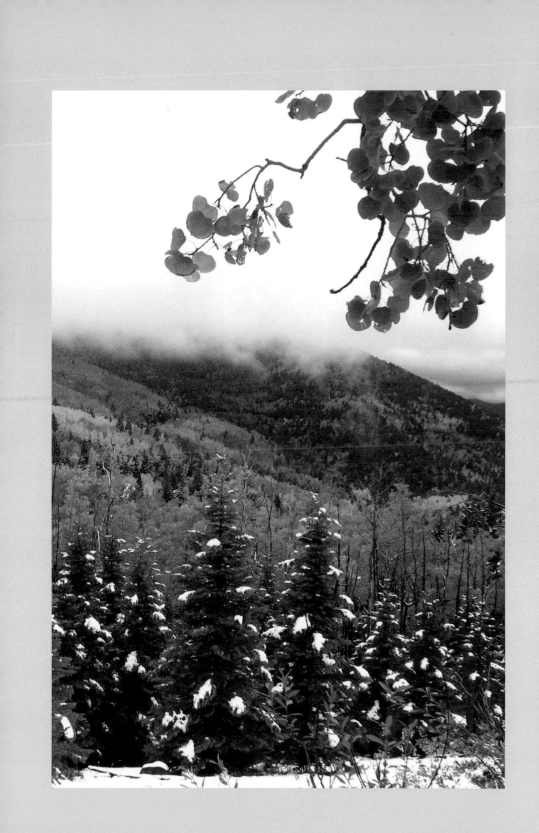

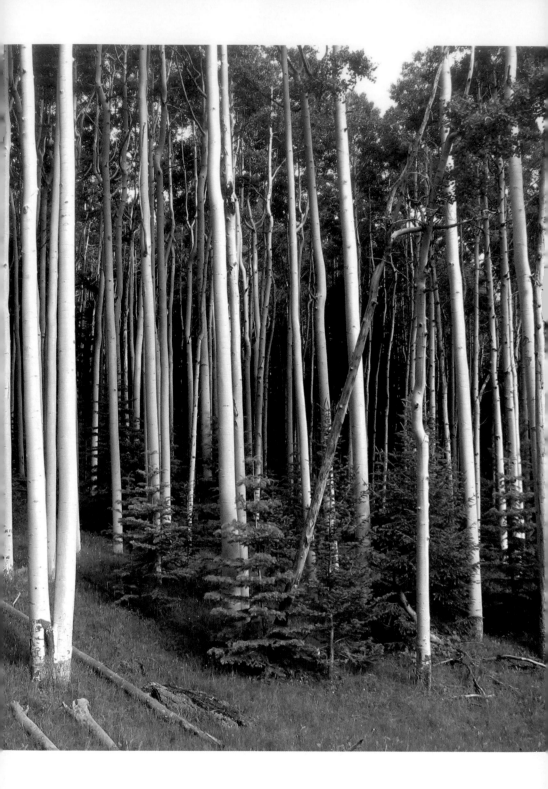

# The Fundamental Framework

**THE FUNDAMENTAL FRAMEWORK** of backpacking governs how we see our equipment and its use. It is an amalgam of many years of trial and error, evolution in equipment, basic economics, and the need to use what we have and can afford. These rules create a lens through which the backpacking equipment world is viewed and used. They create a mindset that is the governing basis for all decisions we make in regard to backcountry gear and how we use it. If we want to enter into the world of ultralight equipment, we must first understand the mindset that governs the framework.

Conventional backpacking has a baseline set of rules:

⚙ No matter what I do, my base weight is heavy—that's to be expected.

⚙ Even with expensive new gear, my base weight will still be more than 20–25 pounds.

⚙ Forty to fifty pounds of weight (often more) is normal for a multiday outing.

⚙ I need a robust pack to carry such weight comfortably.

⚙ A 3-pound pack is really light and may not be comfortable enough to handle such weight.

⚙ A 5- to 6-pound pack is heavy, but it's worth it for the comfort.

So-called "ultralight" gear is flimsy and inappropriate if you want to be comfortable on the trail.

For ultralight backpacking the baseline set of rules is quite different:

 With ultralight gear, backpacking is a series of "conventional day hikes" linked together, since pack weight is the same as or less than conventional day-hike packs.

 Base weight should be less than 10 pounds. A 7- to 9-pound base weight is preferable and achievable.

 Since total pack weight will be 15–25 pounds, a light pack will do the job easily and comfortably.

 To achieve a lower base weight, every ounce counts.

 There must be multiple uses for each piece of gear. This ensures minimal weight with all necessities met.

For those of us traditional backpackers who want to carry less weight, the move to ultralight is a paradigm shift. We must begin to view the entire world of backcountry gear from a new perspective. We will not be successful if we simply buy an ultralight pack and stuff it with conventional gear. Going ultralight, or even in the direction of ultralight, takes serious self-discipline. To succeed, we must focus our efforts and do what it takes to overcome our own backpacking prejudice, our own past ways of being and doing. The basic principles that will guide us through this transition are shown on the following page.

If we can reset our viewpoint and get inspired to carry a fraction of what we're used to, we will be open to exciting new possibilities.

## Basic Principles for Transition

- Make a list of all current expectations and underlying assumptions you have about backpacking gear and backpacking in general. Give yourself permission not to allow these to control your thinking.

- Expect to be surprised.

- Open your mind to new possibilities.

- Be willing to change the way you pack and use your gear.

- Be honest with yourself regarding your comfort needs.

- Be willing to start over with your gear: You may have to replace almost everything so that minimal weight can be achieved.

*Genuine beginnings begin within us, even when they are brought to our attention by external opportunities.*

—William Throsby Bridges

# CHAPTER 1

# Where to Begin?

WHERE TO BEGIN? Well, in truth you have already begun by opening this book, by deciding that you wish to lighten up. The next step is to commit to follow through and do exactly that.

You will need to understand where you are in relation to where you want to be. This means you need to take stock of your gear, and I'll show you how to do that.

What comes next is the part that some find hard to do. To succeed at this you need to look through someone else's eyes to gain a new perspective. This is the required paradigm shift: It's looking through a new set of glasses, a new set of values. The process this creates enables you to look at yourself and your gear from a whole new viewpoint, allowing progress that cannot be attained otherwise.

From this uniquely new perspective you can decide what gear to take, what needs to be replaced, and how best to organize and pack it. I will guide you through this.

Let's begin.

*Once you realize that the road is the goal and that you are always on the road, not to reach a goal, but to enjoy its beauty and its wisdom, life ceases to be a task and becomes natural and simple, in itself an ecstasy.*

—SRI NISARGADATTA MAHARAJ

## The Backpacking Mindset

WE ALL SEE LIFE DIFFERENTLY and hence experience backpacking from very different perspectives. In order to better understand the world of ultralight gear usage, we must first define the arena in which we plan to use this gear. When I teach backpacking classes, I always ask people for their motivation behind the expenditure of time, effort, and money required to participate.

I get wildly varying answers. Each of us needs to be clear on the reason we are using this equipment. What are the priorities?

I asked a friend of mine who has been backcountry skiing, backpacking, hiking, rock climbing, and so on, for more than 60 years what his definition of backpacking is. His answer was revealing:

> *Backpacking is sustained suffering leading to uncomfortable camping with limited gear, in order to do something else.*

This experienced backcountry guy loves the wilderness and uses backpacking as a means to accomplish other goals, like climbing peaks. The backpacking itself is not central.

For me, the journey is at least half of the fun, so my perspective is quite different. Here's my definition:

> *Backpacking is a means to engage the wilderness to experience its richness. It is an opening to extend wonder, see and feel exquisite beauty, explore my inner self, be present in my body, share fantastic silence, do cool things in amazing places, and have fun!*

Our priorities and end-goals truly influence how we approach this game. At this point you should take a few minutes to close this book and write down your goals. Why are you backpacking? What do you want to accomplish? How important is the journey relative to the end goal? What is your definition of backpacking?

Independent of objectives, in order to accomplish our goals we need to take on a special kind of thinking, an attitude that becomes our perspective of wilderness experience. (For those of you new to backpacking, you should know that in addition to this, backpacking requires some basic knowledge in order to be safe and fun.)

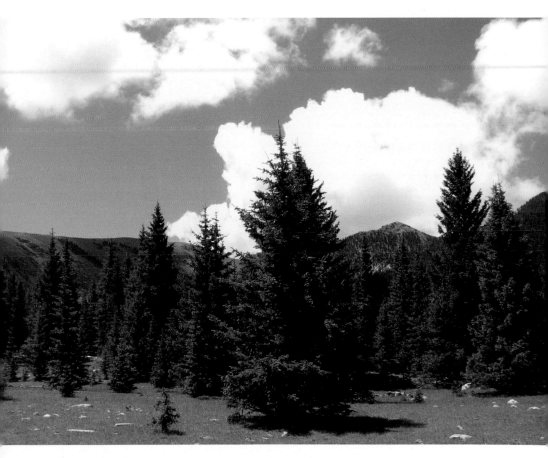

Why am I here?

*To protect what is wild is to protect what is gentle. Perhaps the wilderness we fear is the pause within our own heartbeats, the silent space that says we live only by grace. Wilderness lives by this same grace.*

—TERRY TEMPEST WILLIAMS

# The Ground Rules

THE GROUND RULES for our wilderness-experience attitude form the foundation not only for our thinking, but also for our actions. Once these are established, we can delve into how to achieve goals and what model of backpacking we wish to follow.

## DO NO HARM

My father was a surgeon. He very well knew the principle of "do no harm." He also loved the out-of-doors where his ethic spilled over into our camping trips. There he taught us kids from an early age to respect and appreciate the beauty and fragility of the wilderness. I remember him setting up his huge canvas tent for us to sleep in, being careful not to harm the nearby trees or flowers. His approach still applies today and can be succinctly stated: "Take only pictures; leave only footprints."

These ground rules apply to both conventional and ultralight backpacking. Leave No Trace principles give us the framework for how to do this.

The Leave No Trace concept is more than 50 years old. It was started in the 1960s by the U.S. Forest Service in response to the biophysical effects of increased usage of wilderness public lands.

But it was not until 1994 that the Leave No Trace Center for Outdoor Ethics was incorporated through a joint effort by the National Outdoor Leadership School

(NOLS), the U.S. Forest Service, various federal land management agencies, and outdoor industry and sporting-trade organizations, among others. This nonprofit center, according to its website at **lnt.org,** was established to "develop and expand Leave No Trace training and educational resources, spread the general program components, and engage a diverse range of partners from the federal land management agencies and outdoor industry corporations to non-profit environmental and outdoor organizations and youth-serving groups."

The center came up with seven principles for the ethical use of wild lands. I paraphrase here their copyrighted list:

- ⚙ **Plan ahead and prepare:** Make provisions for extreme weather, hazards, and emergencies; visit in small groups; and split larger parties into groups of four to six.

- ⚙ **Travel and camp on durable surfaces:** Use established trails; use campsites or camp on rock, gravel, dry grasses, or snow, at least 200 feet from water.

- ⚙ **Dispose of waste properly:** Pack it in, pack it out (all trash, leftover food, toilet paper, and litter), deposit solid human waste in catholes dug 6–8 inches deep.

- ⚙ **Leave what you find:** Preserve the past (examine, but do not touch, cultural or historic structures and artifacts); leave rocks, plants, and other natural objects as you find them.

- ⚙ **Minimize campfire impacts:** Campfires can cause lasting impacts; use a lightweight stove for cooking and enjoy a candle lantern for light.

- ⚙ **Respect wildlife:** Observe wildlife from a distance; never feed animals; protect wildlife and your food by storing rations and trash securely; and control pets, or leave them at home.

- ⚙ **Be considerate of other visitors:** Respect other visitors, be courteous; yield to other users on the trail; take breaks and camp away from trails and other visitors; let nature's sounds prevail; and avoid loud voices and noises.

## WHAT OUR PRIORITIES SAY ABOUT US

I want to have fun in the backcountry, and having to give first aid to someone who is injured takes away my fun, so safety has to be my first concern. Hence, it's pretty obvious what my priorities for backpacking must be:

**Safety:** Plan ahead, use common sense, and be flexible.

**Leave no trace:** Show respect for the land and water.

**Have fun:** Show respect for self and others.

**Learn and grow from your experiences:** Be observant, open to wonder, and learn from the mountains and canyons.

Your priorities may differ from mine, but I encourage you to include "Leave no trace" in your list. You may guess what the next question is: Who's responsible for enforcing these priorities? Naturally, of course, we are.

- ❁ **Safety:** We are accountable for our own safety, hygiene, and health. We are also responsible for not putting others at risk through our actions.

- ❁ **Respect:** We are responsible for showing respect: to ourselves (humility and confidence), to others (willingness to give up personal goals for the safety of others), and to the land and water (Leave No Trace principles).

- ❁ **Knowing your limits:** If in doubt, we should ask advice from those with more experience. The wilderness is no place for a big ego!

Once these ground rules are firmly established, setting personal goals, organizing gear, and planning trips become very doable. What gear to take depends on your mindset, how long you will be out, expected weather, the trip objectives, your personal comfort needs, who else is going on the trip and their experience, and possible special needs.

At this point, the first thing we need to consider is what viewpoint we want to assume. We can choose to use conventional gear and its associated mindset, or we can choose the ultralight framework and its gear set, or we can possibly choose a bridge between these two worlds. Those of us experienced in traditional backpacking have an unconscious mindset in place that we need to reconsider if we want to enter the world of the ultralight. This is not insurmountable, but it must be taken into account if we wish to navigate this transition smoothly.

# CHAPTER 2

# The Paradigm Shift

THE ILLUSTRATIONS ON THE NEXT PAGE demonstrate that our viewpoint changes what we see. Our perception dictates which version of each optical illusion we see. Similarly, our viewpoint, based on our values and beliefs, shapes how we think about and implement all backpacking adventures, how we choose and use our gear, and the general approach we take to outdoor adventure.

Beginner backpackers do not have to move from one set of values and beliefs to another to begin backpacking. Experienced backpackers who are used to conventional backpacking equipment and its corresponding thinking will need to experience a paradigm shift in thought and attitudes toward backpacking gear, its usage, and its organization in order to incorporate ultralight ideas.

In the years I've been thinking about ultralight gear, I seem to continually find myself falling into the trap of my old values, old viewpoints, and conventional thinking. This is, of course, the natural result of many years of looking at the world through the same glasses. I'll look at a piece of gear and think, "Of course I need to take that!" Then, if I'm honest with myself, I realize that the reason I want to take it is only that I've always taken it. How can we get out of this holding pattern? The first step to enter a paradigm shift is to confront our own biases, built-in habits, hidden beliefs, and perspectives that form the basis of how we see life.

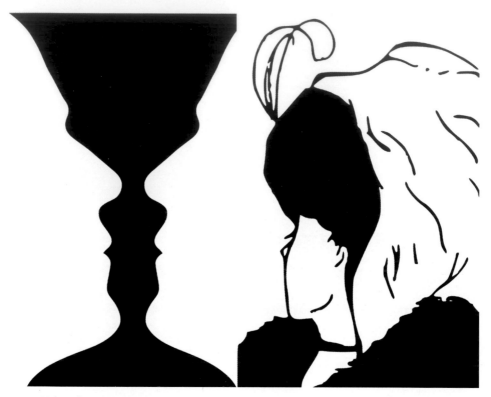

What do you see?

We need to be aware of our mindset and its values before we can shift to another if we so desire. Without this awareness, shifting is either sudden and traumatic, or accidental, and therefore not when we need it. We discussed above some of the central characteristics of the conventional backpacking and ultralight backpacking mental frameworks, along with some suggestions about assumptions as we go through the shift. These will help us in our quest to be free of the habits that limit our transition. Then, as we consider ultralight gear, ultralight attitudes, and ultralight backpacking as a new way of being in the wilderness, we can be aware of the assumptions and expectations in our mind that come from the conventional backpacking world. With this awareness, we can choose to not apply those assumptions in this arena. Then we are free to make decisions that are not based on or biased by such habit-based thinking.

We need to be honest with ourselves about our strengths, weaknesses, and needs. This is especially true in the area of personal comfort. Here is a list of questions that might help:

- How much cushion do you need in your sleeping pad? This will dictate the style of pad you need and available options.

- Do you get cold easily? If so, this might mean you need a warmer sleeping bag and pad, and possibly a down jacket as well. This answer also dictates what clothing layers you will need on each trip.

- Do you need a chair in camp?

- Do you need rain gear? If so, is a rain jacket enough, or do you also need rain pants? If you need rain pants, do they need to be insulated? Do you need non-waterproof insulated pants with rain pants to go over them?

- Do you need bug protection along with rain protection in your shelter? If so, a tarp alone is not enough.

- Where you camp, is the land soft enough for tent stakes, or are there rocks or other natural things that can be used to anchor a non-freestanding tent? If not, you might need a freestanding shelter.

- What kind of cooking do you plan to do? Size of pot(s) and the specific kind of stove to bring are dependent upon this answer. Are you cooking for only yourself or also for others?

- Do you have specific dietary needs that dictate specific foods and ways of cooking?

- What water sources are available where you backpack? Is there the possibility of human feces in the water? Is the water clear or murky? Is it deep or running, or just a pothole with a bit of water in it? These dictate the type of water purification or filtration system you bring.

- Are there water sources en route, so you can carry only a small amount of water and refill along the way? Or do you need to carry water for the entire trek?

- Have you hiked in low-cut lightweight hiking shoes or trail-running shoes? Do you need heavy hiking boots if your pack is only 20 pounds?

How much of a first-aid kit do you really need? Are you the doctor for a large group, or just needing to cover possible injuries for yourself? How likely is it that you will encounter an injured party en route or need to help someone else in your own group?

 How often do you actually use a knife or multiuse tool in the backcountry? How many uses does the tool you take need to have? Would a razor blade suffice?

 Some people bring a lot of clothes when backpacking. Could you get by with just one change of underwear and a clean pair of socks?

 Do you tend to lose gear on trips? Do you have a method of organizing your gear?

All of these and other such questions help us refine our gear choices. If we are not honest with our answers, we will probably find we are unhappy with decisions based on those answers.

 ## Quick Tips

✓ Consider what you do habitually when you backpack. Now consider why you do these things.

✓ Look honestly at how you think about backpacking gear. What are your expectations?

*Your problem is to bridge the gap that exists between where you are now and the goal you intend to reach.*

—EARL NIGHTINGALE

# The Concept of Bridging

BEFORE WE GET TOO DEEP into specifics, I want to acknowledge the spectrum of available gear choices. Take a look at the diagram below. On one extreme, we find the zealous conventional backpacker who carries whatever is desired regardless of weight, resulting in very heavy and bulky loads that are easily more than 60 pounds for a weeklong trip. At the other extreme are the thru-hiking ultra-ultralight backpackers who are meticulously careful about every gram of weight, resulting in extremely light loads in the range of 10–15 pounds for a weeklong trip. Along this spectrum of gear choices are wide differences in comfort, multiuse, contingency planning, gear organization, temperature and weather preparedness, and willingness to endure adverse conditions with minimal protection, along with attitudes and goals. Where are you today on this spectrum? Where would you like to be?

**Spectrum of Gear Choices: Example Weights for a Weeklong Trip**

| Under 15 Pounds | 25–30+ Pounds | 40–50+ Pounds | 60+ Pounds |
|---|---|---|---|
| Ultra-Ultralight | Bridging Gear | Average Conventional | Zealous Conventional |

In order to transition from average conventional gear usage to a lighter-weight approach that preserves comfort and contingency preparedness, most of us cannot simply jump from one extreme to the other. I certainly could not! For me, personal comfort is very important, so I decided it was OK for me to trade off some weight for my own needs. Backpacking is, after all, for fun!

My own experience dictated that I explore gear that I call "bridge" gear, ultralight-like gear that is more like conventional gear than strict ultralight gear, and that is more comfortable and easier to use. It is gear that bridges between ultralight and conventional approaches. These types of gear enable an easier transition and more effective selection, leading to successful and fun backpacking that is much lighter than the conventional approach but heavier and more full-service than the strict ultralight approach.

For example, the backpacks that worked best for me include such "extras" as load-lifters, ergonomic hip belts, a bit more padding and breathability in the back-plane of the pack, and ergonomically cut shoulder straps. Although common on conventional backpacks, many ultralight packs do not include these. The weight for such bridge packs ranges from 10 to 14 ounces heavier than the ultralight equivalents. The pure ultralight approach for shelters might include only a tarp, where the bridge shelters include more weather coverage, bug protection, and some sort of ground cloth.

Before we go through categories of equipment, in which I will be sharing how I arrived at the bridge solutions that saved me considerable weight, we must first understand where we are now.

  ## Quick Tips

✓ The trick to lighter gear and an overall lighter pack is to reconsider what you really need for comfortable backpacking.

✓ As a conventional backpacker, you don't have to take on the values of the ultralighter; you just need to learn from their approach. This means you need to consider a new way of thinking.

*Toto, I have a feeling we're not in Kansas anymore.*

—L. FRANK BAUM

## CHAPTER 3

# Understanding Where We Are Now

WE BEGIN BY ASSESSING where we are and where we've been in the field of backcountry gear so we can understand what has to change. This applies not only to our gear, but also to our bodies. Ever notice that ultralight backpackers are all skinny, strong, and fit? If we're shaving ounces off our packs, we should also be sure we're not carrying extra pounds on our bodies. A healthy body weight will help ensure we use minimal effort when hiking and backpacking.

Many of us have been lightening our packs for a number of years, so not everything in our quiver of equipment needs to be replaced. We now need to take an inventory of what gear we consider essential, find out what it weighs, and decide how important it is to us personally on any given trip. This inventory is also a pathway to minimize frustration through logical organization of our gear.

Let's start by considering how to collect our gear.

# Gear Organization

MOST OF US are familiar with the concept of the Ten Essentials. This is a list of 10 things that would enable you to survive an unexpected overnight in any outdoor condition. (Notice I said survive, not enjoy.) Developed in the 1930s from an organization called, appropriately, The Mountaineers, the list has morphed over time into any number of combinations, but here is a version that is pretty common today:

- ⚙ **Extra clothing:** extra socks, gloves, insulated pants, jacket, rain gear, warm hat

- ⚙ **Fire:** fire starter and matches (storm-proof or in a watertight container)

- ⚙ **First aid:** first-aid kit, insulating pad, pencil and paper, signal mirror, whistle

- ⚙ **Hydration:** water bottle or reservoir and treatment method

- ⚙ **Illumination:** headlamp or flashlight (with extra batteries)

- ⚙ **Navigation:** map and compass plus trail description (optional: GPS, altimeter)

- ⚙ **Nutrition:** energy bars, gels, or food for one extra day

- ⚙ **Repair:** cord, duct tape, fabric-repair tape, knife (or multiuse tool), needle and thread, safety pins, wire

- ⚙ **Shelter:** emergency bivvy (bivouac sack) or tarp

- ⚙ **Sun protection:** sun hat, sunglasses, sunscreen (SPF 15–30)

## MODULAR PACKING SYSTEMS BASED ON THE TEN ESSENTIALS

My experience has been that it is better to organize my gear into "systems" of like items, logically co-locating those items used together rather than simply gathering them up. When I pack for a trip, the gear for each system is packed into one stuff sack (with the possible exception of the shelter and sleeping system, because conventionally it's too big to fit in one sack and balances better in the pack if it is divided into separate pieces). I recommend organizing gear into the following modular packing systems:

- Hiking System (things worn, not packed, like your pack and trekking poles, boots, and so on)

- Clothing System

- Shelter, Sleeping and Lighting System

- Navigation System

- First-Aid, Repair, and Personal-Hygiene System

- Communication System

- Fire System

- Nutrition System

- Specialty-Gear System

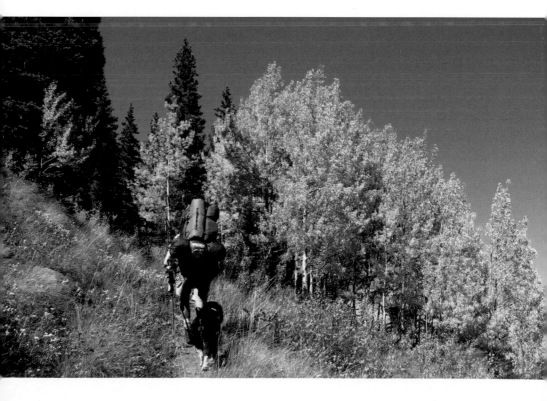

Within these nine systems, everything you need to take on any given trip can be organized. We will discuss these systems in more detail later. The list of items within each system is not static. It may change from one trip to the next depending on the requirements of each trip. Create a new gear list for each trip. Over time, this will create a master list that includes items most used. Each new trip will take some subset of the master list. Use a process to generate your gear lists based on what you need to accomplish on each trip. ("Packing to Minimize Frustration," page 122, provides more details on how to pack your gear.)

## CREATING GEAR LISTS THAT WORK

To create a gear list for any given trip, use the simple steps listed on the following page. This will be different for each trip, and it needs to be done before each trip. Experiment until you create the gear lists that work best for your trips. Get to know your personal preferences and comfort levels necessary for safety and happiness. Then choose gear that meets these needs while minimizing weight. Take only what you need. Certainly after doing this a few times you will find a central core list of items needed on most trips. This process ensures you have what you need without carrying extra weight.

 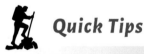 *Quick Tips*

✓ Packing modularly in a logical way minimizes frustration in the backcountry, helps us find gear quickly, and helps us not lose things inadvertently. Using the Ten Essentials as the framework to do this not only makes sense, it ensures we have everything we need for both comfort and safety.

✓ Creating gear lists by understanding the functions we need to perform on each individual trip minimizes the weight we carry while ensuring we can do everything we need to do, including contingencies.

The table beginning on page 32 shows my master gear list. I've used it again and again for a number of Grand Canyon treks (using conventional gear). It shows how to organize the gear based on the Ten Essentials and is now a refined list for those specific kinds of trips. You should create your own lists based on your own kinds of trips. Even with this list in place, I always take a subset of it on each specific trip, never the entire list.

## How to Create a Gear List

- ✷ List the functions you need to do on this trip.

- ✷ Pick the gear best suited for each function.

- ✷ Take only what you need.

- ✷ Refine your gear list based on the following:

    - ◇ *where you will be going,*

    - ◇ *what time of year it is,*

    - ◇ *possible contingency situations, and*

    - ◇ *the expected weather conditions.*

# Example Multiday Grand Canyon Trek Personal-Equipment List

### 1. HIKING SYSTEM:

- ✱ 30-foot cord, bear bag or stuff sack, extra straps, and so on
- ✱ Backcountry permit attached to pack
- ✱ Boots
- ✱ Camelbak bladder and collapsible water bottles (for hiking and in camp)
- ✱ Chair or pad (for lunches and evenings and meditation)
- ✱ Clothes to hike in (hanky, pants, shirt, socks, sunglasses, sun hat, underwear)
- ✱ Pack
- ✱ Rain cover for pack, and extra trash bags
- ✱ Rain gear (see Clothing System)
- ✱ Trekking poles

### 2. CLOTHING SYSTEM:

- ✱ Down jacket
- ✱ Extra underwear, extra hiking socks, camp socks
- ✱ Hats (baseball and winter), gloves, neck gaiter
- ✱ Insulated pants
- ✱ Mid-layer jacket
- ✱ Rain coat and pants
- ✱ Sleeping clothes

### 3. SHELTER, SLEEPING, AND LIGHTING SYSTEM:

- ✱ Headlamp and extra batteries, and/or extra headlamp
- ✱ Pee bottle

❁ Sleeping bag, stuff sack, bag liner (if needed for extra warmth), pillow or pillow case, ear plugs

❁ Sleeping pad

❁ Tent (including tent body, fly, footprint, stakes, poles)

### 4. NAVIGATION SYSTEM:

❁ Compass, contingency plans, GPS (if needed), maps, route descriptions

### 5. FIRST-AID, REPAIR, AND PERSONAL-HYGIENE SYSTEM:

❁ Bug repellent (as necessary), lotion, sunscreen

❁ First-aid kit

❁ Personal medicines

❁ Repair and contingency kit (duct tape, emergency bivvy, extra straps, safety pins, sewing kit, wire)

❁ Tiny towel

❁ Toiletries (hand sanitizer, toilet paper, toothbrush, tooth powder, washcloth)

❁ Zip-top plastic bags (for packing out used toilet paper)

### 6. COMMUNICATION SYSTEM:

❁ Signal mirror, whistle (contingency as needed)

❁ Two-way radios (if warranted)

### 7. FIRE SYSTEM:

❁ Cooking pot(s)

❁ Emergency fire starter (steel wool); knife, multiuse tool, or razor blade; pocket lighter (such as Bic), waterproof matches, and so on

❁ Stove and fuel

## Example Multiday Grand Canyon Trek Personal-Equipment List (continued)

**8. NUTRITION SYSTEM:**

- ⚙ Breakfasts
- ⚙ Camp snacks, libations, etc.
- ⚙ Desserts (as desired)
- ⚙ Dinners and soups
- ⚙ Energy bars and hiking snacks (chocolate, ginger, nuts, trail mix, and so on)
- ⚙ Lunches
- ⚙ Spoon and cup
- ⚙ Tea and other drinks
- ⚙ Water filter or Aquamira water-treatment drops (and bucket with alum if needed)

**9. SPECIALTY-GEAR SYSTEM:**

- ⚙ Canyoneering-specific gear
- ⚙ Climbing harness (or Alpine Bod harness), and climbing-specific gear
- ⚙ Climbing or canyoneering rope(s)
- ⚙ Climbing shoes
- ⚙ Hand-line rope(s)

"*C*ontrariwise," continued Tweedledee, "if it was so, it might be; and if it were so, it would be; but as it isn't, it ain't. That's logic."

— Lewis Carroll

## GEAR ASSESSMENT

Make a list of all of your gear using the above categories as a way to assess what you own now. Some items may fall into more than one category (for example, hiking system *and* clothing system). That's OK, just put the items in the list where they most make sense to you.

Once you have the list made, start a spreadsheet with all items listed by system. Go through the gear one item at a time, weighing each item with a food scale.

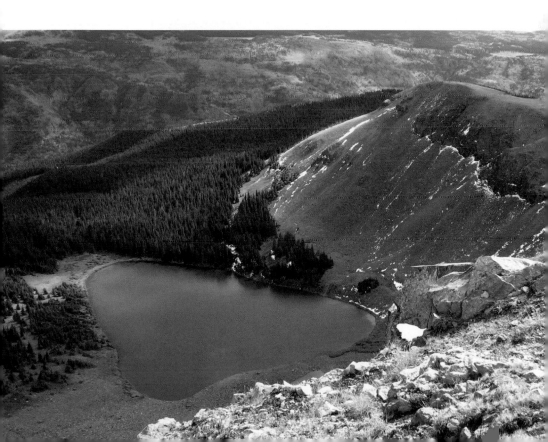

Use something that will measure accurately in grams or to 0.1 ounce. Write down the weight by each item in the list. Do this for all of your gear.

If you are beginning in backpacking, make a list of the gear you think you should purchase, rather than what you own. This process can be used to help you decide if ultralight is right for you.

Organize the spreadsheet with the following topics entered in bold across the top row:

1. System Name

2. Item

3. Conventional Weight

4. Replacement Choice

5. Replacement Weight

6. Replacement Cost

7. Weight Savings

8. Importance Rating

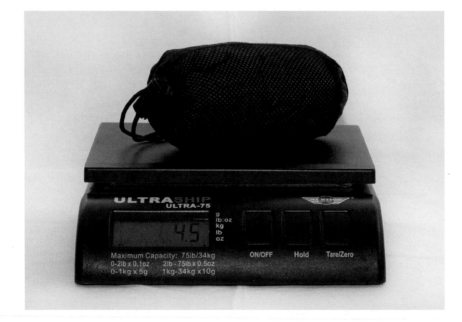

A kitchen scale works well for weighing gear.

Fill in the table with the data for your conventional gear, based on what you just measured. Keep all items in each gear system listed together, and enter a blank row between systems to make it easier to read. Don't worry for now about the replacement items. If you are savvy with Excel, you can set it up to sum the weights at the bottom of the page, or even between systems (summing each system alone). This can be helpful to give you perspective.

The Importance Rating is a guess at how useful, necessary, and important to the success of your backpacking trip the item is. Rate each item from one to 10, with 10 being imperative, one being fluff that is nice to have, or possibly just to have along in case you might need it.

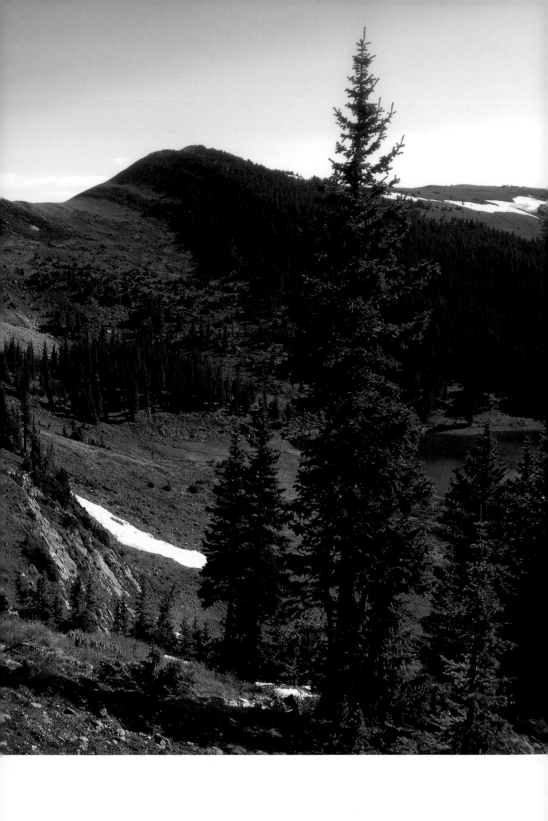

CHAPTER **4**

# Recontextualizing Each Gear System

LET'S NOW CONSIDER EACH GEAR SYSTEM IN TURN. The objective is to see each one from a new perspective, namely, the mindset of ultralight backpacking tempered by conventional experience and the desire to preserve comfort.

As you read each section in this chapter, consider the following method of reframing your thinking:

Once the mindsets of both kinds of gear are well understood, it is pretty straightforward to replace existing gear with appropriate ultralight substitutes. This does not have to be a radical event. Nor does it have to be expensive, although it can be. My experience here is that it is not effective to look through the eyes of a conventional backpacker when buying ultralight gear. Instead, you must

- decide very carefully what your needs and goals are,

- adopt the attitude of an ultralight backpacker to work toward those specific goals, and

- remember the points listed in "Basic Principles for Transition" (page 13), let go of your established assumptions, and make no new ones.

Now let's look at each system of gear through the window of bridging and consider how to make it lighter and more comfortable.

*In every walk with nature one receives far more than he seeks.*

—JOHN MUIR

## The Hiking System

THIS SYSTEM IS what is worn or carried, not packed. This gear system is just as important as the contents inside the pack, but it is often not mentioned. It includes items like hiking shoes or boots, trekking poles, the pack itself and its rain cover, and the hiking clothes you wear. Rain gear is sometimes included here, but you should list it where it makes most sense to you. Often a hat is included here, but it also can be listed with clothing. Sunglasses can be included here as well. All of these things should be categorized according to how you use your gear. There are no right or wrong ways to list gear.

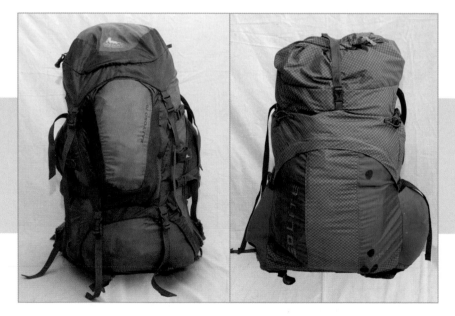

My Conventional Pack
(70-liter Gregory Baltoro)

My Bridge Pack
(50-liter GoLite Jam)

## PACKS

First and foremost in this system is the backpack itself. Conventional thinking expects the load to be heavy, the trail long, and the energy expenditure high. The pack needs to be especially well designed to carry heavy loads, and to be comfortable for long treks with heavy weight. My conventional pack weighs 5.5 pounds, 6 if you include the rain cover. That's 6 pounds of infrastructure to give me comfort on the trail for the 45-pound loads I've traditionally carried. On the other hand, the ultralight back-packer expects to be carrying less than 20 pounds, so carrying it takes little effort, it's always fun, and less energy is expended while hiking. It also means the pack does not need to be especially fancy, padded, technical, or supportive.

Let's begin with how to find the right pack. Seems simple, but I found it more complex than I assumed. Wait, did I just say, "assumed?" Hmmmm, assumptions again!

It seems obvious how to choose a pack: Just search the Internet for the lightest weight and maybe the most popular model, and buy that. Well, that approach might work for some, but it did not work for me. One of my baseline premises in this book is to preserve comfort. That means I have expectations that the pack I choose will be comfortable for me to carry while hiking with the gear I need.

After an online analysis of many packs, I field-tested a number of ultralight packs and several packs that fall into the category of bridge packs. Bridge packs are heavier than ultralight packs, more comfortable in general, sometimes with more features. They are still much lighter than the conventional alternatives while including some of the characteristics that make conventional packs user-friendly. (For testing, I purchased these packs, tested them on day hikes, and then returned all but one of them.)

The ultralight packs I considered weigh from 18 to 28 ounces, while the bridge packs tested weigh from 27 to 40 ounces. I took each of these on a long day hike filled with 25 pounds. I really wanted the 18-ounce pack to be my pick, but I found it too minimal in features, extremely hot on my body (shoulders, chest, back, and hips), and just OK in comfort. The next one up in weight was much more comfortable, and I really liked the fit, but it was also extremely hot on my back; so much so that I found I could not justify calling it comfortable. It did have more features, including an inflatable pad for the back support.

So I began to look for packs that had some way to handle heat and moisture on one's back. This means my comfort was dictating more features, meaning
heavier packs. This began my search for ultralight packs that were more conventional in nature. Such packs are bridge packs, not ultralight. Although I endeav-
ored to enter the ultralight mindset, my requirements for comfort dictated that I
loosen my stringency in choices. This not only opened the door for many more
pack choices, but it also helped me realize how one must transition from conventional to ultralight gear. Here is the process for choosing a pack (the same process
also applies to each category of gear):

- Make a list of all packs under a specific weight (say 1.5 pounds in this case) that are sized appropriately (in volume) for your needs.

- Pick the lightest one and try it out. (For packs, this means taking a hike with the pack full of 25 pounds of gear, for at least five hours of hiking in rough terrain. Do the same hike with the same weight for each candidate pack.)

- Does it meet your comfort needs? If it meets your needs, you're done. If not, figure out what is missing and why it is not meeting your needs. This tells you what to look for in the next round of tests. Iterate through the list until you find one that works or the list is exhausted.

- Exhausted list means your comfort requirements are now dictating that you consider heavier packs. Hence, make the lower weight limit what your upper one has been, and increase the upper weight limit (in this case, 1.5 pounds becomes the lower limit, 2.5 pounds the upper limit).

- Fill in the list with candidate packs using the new weight limits, and iterate on those until you find the lightest one that meets your needs.

Don't worry about how involved and possibly expensive the above process
seems. It can be very simple and fast, or it can be longer and more complex. The
above steps give you the optimal solution in a straightforward way, but it can be
more expensive and take more time if your requirements are to find the very best
pack for your needs. An alternative and simpler approach is to pick the lightest
one on the list and try it out. This will show you what's important to you by what's
missing, or what works and what doesn't. Then pick the lightest pack from the list
that includes the features you need and go with that.

## Quick Tips

✓ The pack is the basis for comfortable hiking. Choose wisely. Make sure it fits well and is adjusted properly.

✓ Remember that one pack may not meet all requirements for all of the kinds of trips you do, so you may need more than one pack if your trips vary significantly in season and gear needs.

✓ To lighten up your pack, begin with a much simpler and lighter pack than you are used to. It should meet your needs without diminishing your comfort.

There are some conventional packs that are lighter than most, but are still relatively heavy packs (in comparison to ultralight). Some of these have a trampoline-mesh back support and other nice features. These are well designed in general, but most weigh in around 40–50 ounces or more, which is out of the range of ultralight. Most of the lighter-weight bridge packs come in around 2 pounds in weight. My bridge pack search began to focus on packs around 28–34 ounces, with more standard features that serve comfort (for example, pockets on the hip belt, functional load lifters, form-fitted hip and shoulder padding, and some way to keep my back, hips, and shoulders cooler). I found this group of packs to be much more familiar in fit and comfort, while still saving me significant weight. (I settled on a 28-ounce bridge pack. It's comfortable, has nice features, and although not 18 ounces, saves me almost 4 pounds from my conventional pack!) Amazing what a few more ounces of comfort can do!

Ultralight backpackers consider "a few more ounces" to be the wrong attitude. However, those of us who know and love conventional backpacking might need a transition—a bridge—from conventional backpacking gear toward ultralight. The result will not be a base weight of 8.5 pounds. But it will be a base weight that is some dozen or more pounds lighter than what we have been carrying! We "transitioners" just need to be sure we don't make that "just a few ounces" into a mantra. It's OK for one or two important items (like packs and sleeping pads, perhaps), but it is not appropriate for everything.

Pack volume is also a consideration. Conventional weeklong trips often require a 65- to 70-liter pack or even larger volume for winter trips. However, ultralight gear usually takes up less space and hence we might easily be able to do a weeklong trip with a smaller volume pack. This will be determined by the total gear collection and how it is packed, whether or not warm layers are included (since down jackets, et al., can be bulky to pack), and if specific extra items are required for a specific trip (like snowshoes, for example). In my case, I tested both 70-liter and 50-liter versions of the same bridge pack, and chose the 50-liter pack. It works well for weeklong trips as long as I don't need to take specialty gear, like climbing gear. (See "The Specialty-Gear System," page 91, for more information.)

Rain covers can be purchased for both conventional and ultralight packs. Some are lighter than others. And certainly one can save weight by replacing the pack rain cover with a plastic bag used to line the inside of the pack. A trash

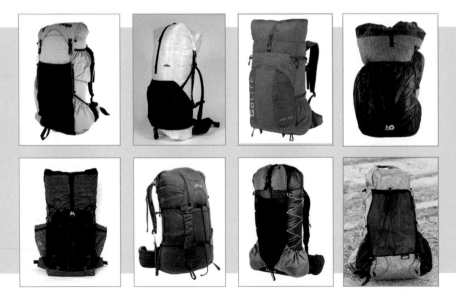

What features do you need in your ultralight pack?

compactor bag works well, size 68 liters and white in color (making it easier to see things inside). It fits nicely inside the pack and encloses everything. This approach allows the pack to get wet in a storm while keeping everything else dry. However, I sometimes use the pack as part of my sleeping system as padding under my feet, so if it gets soaked, that's not so good. So I needed to choose between a commercially purchased lightweight pack cover and an upside-down plastic bag used outside the pack by simply cutting slits in it to allow the shoulder straps to poke out. The latter approach is more ultralight, but not very abrasion resistant.

## TREKKING POLES

Trekking poles are invaluable in conventional backpacking, especially on steep terrain with a full pack. In the ultralight world, they are also important, but for different reasons. Yes, they still help in hiking, and they still offer balance and everything they do for conventional backpackers. But now their use on steep terrain is less necessary since the pack is so much lighter. More to the point, however, they now double as tent poles. And, in the ultralight world, ease of adjustability is paramount, especially inside a tent. Hence, the cam-type trekking poles are a better choice than the twist-type. The cams make them easier to adjust and lock in place quickly when setting up the tent and for adjusting tension in the tent afterward.

It's also key to know ahead of time how and when you will be using these poles on the trek, so you don't get your tent set up and then realize you need the

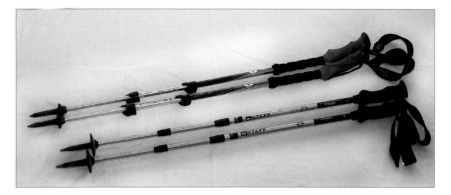

Twist-Style vs. Cam-Style Trekking Poles

poles for a hike from the base camp. If you plan to hike with the poles on day hikes, you must plan ahead for your tent during those times. Obviously, you can collapse the tent; but if you want it upright, you need to bring tent poles, or hike without the trekking poles on these day hikes. Some ultralight tents use only one pole, so one pole stays while one goes hiking.

We'll discuss footwear in the next section, "The Clothing System," even though boots also are considered part of the Hiking System. When a number of layers are taken, the Clothing System becomes necessary as a separate entity. If all you take is what you wear, then the Hiking System and Clothing System become one system. Remember, these systems exist only to help with packing gear and to simplify gear organization. You define what systems you want to use.

I tried on the farmer's hat,

Didn't fit . . .

A little too small—just a bit

Too floppy.

Couldn't get used to it,

Took it off . . .

I tried on the summer sun,

Felt good.

Nice and warm—knew it would.

Tried the grass beneath bare feet,

Felt neat.

Finally, finally felt well dressed,

Nature's clothes fit me best.

—SHEL SILVERSTEIN

# The Clothing System

OF COURSE, layering is the key to effective use of clothing in wilderness activities. I use the four layers listed below, but you should find the right system that works best for your metabolism and activities. Some people use additional layers, some fewer. It all depends on how hot or cold you get, what you eat, the weather conditions, the activities at the time, and specific needs. Moisture management directly impacts body-temperature regulation. Hence, wicking fabrics are imperative for the base layer and often even for the mid-layer, and breathability is central.

The principles behind layering include the maintenance of core temperature, maximizing comfort, and the wise management of skin moisture and temperature. In summary, the layers for three-season backpacking are these:

⚙  wicking base layer: non-cotton T-shirt or long-sleeve base layer

⚙  wicking and warmer mid-layer: often windproof but not waterproof; fleece, down, or synthetic, or possibly just a nylon shell with microfleece inside

⚙  warmer outer layer: down puffy or the like, again not waterproof but much warmer and sized to fit over base layer and mid-layer (Lighter or even ultra-light down jackets or synthetics work for three-season use.)

⚙  waterproof rain shell: waterproof, breathable, windproof, very lightweight, uninsulated outer shell with a hood that fits over all other layers

This list covers layers above the waist. Below the waist can be layered with just underwear, pants, and possibly rain pants. For three-season treks I wear versatile zip-off nylon hiking pants that convert to shorts. They are tough, lightweight, and dry quickly. The zip-off feature allows easy crossing of streams or cooling off when very hot, or even just venting by opening the zips a bit when leg protection is needed but it's warm out. Rain pants over these allow layering for inclement conditions, along with insulated pants for shoulder-season treks.

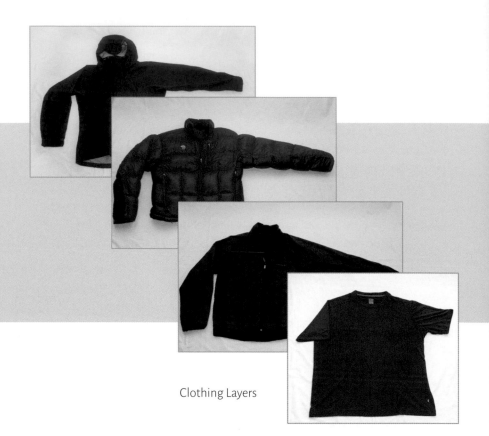

Clothing Layers

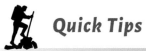 ## Quick Tips

✓ The key to layering is moisture management combined with flexibility to handle many kinds of weather.

✓ Choose clothes that fit for the layer they represent. That is, skin layer might fit snugly, but the rain shell should be loose enough to fit over a number of other layers. Each layer piece must fit according to its expected use.

## LAYERS UPON LAYERS

For ultralight configurations, the difference from conventional layering will be in the specifics of the layers themselves. Conventional backpackers want lightweight gear, but they are, in general, more interested in great functionality. That is, each layer must perform well for its specific purpose. In the ultralight world, lightest weight comes first, and functionality must include multipurpose use (that is, each garment must work for more than one thing). Hence, where we might use a 16-ounce rain coat in conventional trekking because it fits well, has pit zips, is super-durable for bushwhacking through brush, and is waterproof and very breathable, for ultralight rain gear, we seek ones that are less than 9 ounces for each piece (coat and pants), waterproof, and breathable, and we understand that these are not as durable and might not be as breathable or adjustable as conventional choices.

There are many nice coats in the 12- to 18-ounce range, but few in the lighter weights that are fully functional. Some ultralighters may be OK with one that is not very breathable that comes in at 8 ounces. My lightweight raincoat weighs 6.2 ounces and is fully functional as rain protection, but it is not as warm or windproof as my 17-ounce conventional jacket (that I use in the winter), nor is it anywhere close to being tough enough to handle serious bushwhacking (more on this below). But for the rare times here in the Southwest that we have rain, it is perfect. A compromise for increased wind and bushwhacking protection is to pick a shell in the 9- to 10-ounce range.

I found some rain pants that are only 2.9 ounces (for a size medium)! These are definitely not breathable, but they are very functional and unbelievably light. They are expensive because they are made out of Cuben Fiber, and they're not easy to put on over boots because they have no zippers or anything to help with that, but they do the job. My argument for these is that if rain comes only once in a blue moon, carrying the dead weight of an unused rain pant most of the time is a great reason to buy something less than 3 ounces. At these lower weights, don't expect a full side zipper in rain pants. Such a zip on the side allows for venting as well as ease of putting on/taking off over hiking boots. I find I really enjoy having a full zip on the side because much of my hiking and trekking is in the Southwest, where rainstorms last a short time, clear up, and then come back for short spells. Venting between storms is easier and nicer than taking the pants off only to re-don

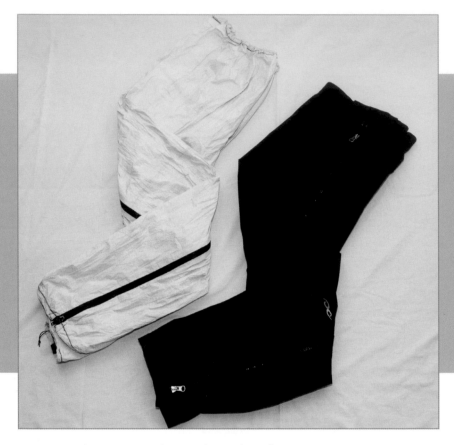

Conventional rain pants are heavier than Cuben Fiber rain pants.

them a few minutes later. My older full-zip rain pants have been great, but are heavy by these standards. So, for 2.9 ounces, the Cuben Fiber is worth considering, and I recently added side zips to mine at only an ounce increase in weight. I just have to be careful with them when bushwhacking, as the fabric is not as durable as the heavier standards.

I should note that durability is a trade-off with ultralight fabrics. Those of us who enjoy bushwhacking as part of our outdoor activities will notice that ultralight rain jackets and pants do weigh much less, but they are also much less durable in the face of rugged terrain, thorns, bushes, tree branches, and thickets through which bushwhacking often takes us. (The same is true for packs and tents as well.) In addition, although fully rainproof and breathable, many of these ultralight rain jackets are not as windproof as their heavier sisters. This plays into their ability to provide warmth as the outermost layer of our layering system. As mentioned above, sometimes it may be appropriate to carry a heavier rain shell to handle the weather and temperatures expected, especially in winter.

## SLEEP-SYSTEM CLOTHING

Another ultralight layering concept is using clothing as part of the sleep system. For many ultralighters, outerwear garments form part of the methodology for keeping warm at night. Some people bring a superlight sleeping bag or quilt, and bundle up in all of the clothing layers at night. Again, this has to do with minimum weight, which dictates multiple uses for each gear item.

If you are a "cold sleeper" (get cold easily), as I am, this method is my ace in the hole (rather than using clothes as my primary warmth element in the sleep system) for when the planned sleeping arrangement fails to keep me warm and I need to add layers in the middle of the night. However, everyone can use this approach if the warmth of the clothing layers is included in the calculation of how warm your sleeping system will keep you. The layers I'm discussing here are things like a mid-layer and down puffy, along with insulated pants. Under these, a base layer separate from what you hike in works best. This allows you to sleep in dry, clean clothes while your body heat dries the damp shirt and socks of the day in the foot of the sleeping bag. This is a matter of personal taste. Some folks like to wear one set of clothes all day long and all night, too. Part of my comfort-bridging is that my sleeping clothes are dedicated for that—cotton skivvies and a wicking shirt at night, and all wicking fabrics during the day. And I have found that sleeping in a damp, and possibly dirty, hiking shirt is not very comfortable, so it's nice to have something specifically for sleeping.

In the new system, this is a trade-off of a few ounces for the comfort this shirt provides (and it acts as a backup for my daytime base-layer shirt). In cold weather it's no trade-off, because I use long underwear to sleep in rather than my cold, and sometimes wet, clothes. I can put layers over the underwear if it's really cold (for example, during winter camping). In all cases, my damp socks and shirt from today's hiking go into the sleeping bag at the foot of the bag. This dries them overnight and makes them warm to put on in the cool of early morning. And I always have extra pairs of dry socks.

The trade-offs between down, hydrophobic down, and synthetic sleeping bags apply here also. Down is lighter weight and more compressible than synthetic for a given warmth (usually). This, of course, depends on the quality of the down and the quality of the synthetic. Good quality down will last some 30 years if well maintained; synthetic insulation can be expected to last 7–10 years. The higher the quality of the down (higher fill number—for example, 850–1,000), the more compressible and lighter weight it is for a given warmth, and, of course, more expensive. These qualities apply to down sleeping bags, quilts, and clothing (jackets, pants, and vests) equally. We'll talk more about down and sleeping systems later (see "The Shelter, Sleeping, and Lighting System," on page 56). Here, it is simply important to know that more options become available by coordinating clothing layers with whatever your sleeping system includes.

Insulated pants are often part of these options and are another trade-off that affects some of us. Evenings and mornings can be cold in camp (as can winter camping in general). So in addition to normal rain pants, extra insulation for legs is important, especially if you get cold easily and like to backpack in country where the rain is cold. Some insulated pants are waterproof but heavier. These could replace rain pants while offering warmth. Other insulated pants are light but not waterproof, only water-resistant. So you must choose which meets your needs for the most trips. Obviously, if your trips are in the Northwest or Southeast of the

 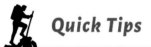

## Quick Tips

✓ Insulated layers that will be used as part of the sleeping system must work in all weather conditions. Unless you are willing to tolerate wet clothes inside your sleeping bag, insulated layers must be protected from rain by other layers.

✓ The choice of whether or not to use clothes as part of the sleeping system depends not only on weight and comfort, but also on the season, altitude, duration, weather, and contingencies of each specific trip.

continental United States, synthetic waterproof pants would be best due to the high humidity and rain potential. In the high-altitude and desert areas of Arizona, Colorado, New Mexico, and Utah, lighter down alternatives work fine, especially if ultralight rain pants are available to layer over them when necessary. Again, some pants have side zips that allow easier donning and venting, but they are generally heavier than those without zippers. When they are part of your sleeping system, the weight is justified, but they might not work so well as part of the sleeping system if they are soaked from a long day hiking in the rain. So, as you may have guessed, choosing rain pants along with insulated pants, or selecting only one of these, is another trade-off for personal comfort.

## HAPPY FEET, HAPPY TRIP

The last thing in clothing we need to consider is footwear. Your feet are an essential part of your arsenal, so take good care of them. Without happy feet, no trip will be fun. For conventional backpacks, I've worn out a variety of boots over the years, many brands and styles. In recent years I have found boots made by Zamberlan (handcrafted full-leather boots made in Italy) are pretty light in weight (3.5 pounds per pair), are very comfortable, give no blisters, provide great ankle and arch support, and handle extremely rough terrain easily. Over the years I've learned that it doesn't really matter what others wear; it matters what fits my feet! So for me, this has been a superior solution for many happy Grand Canyon treks and trips up Colorado 14ers. Now as I enter the world of ultralight gear, the question arises, do I need these boots? My trail-hiker shoes weigh only 2 pounds, 3 ounces, and many new trail-running shoes are lighter yet. Will they work for backpacking instead of my boots when I'm carrying so much less?

I have a friend who is a trail runner. He wears his tattered super-lightweight trail-running shoes on all of our conventional backpacking trips, while I'm in my (relatively heavy) boots. The ultralight approach is never to wear heavy boots, because the pack weighs so little (less than 20 pounds). What's important here is "what works for your feet." I have high arches, so I need orthotics, which make any foot gear more comfortable for me and minimize foot fatigue. I use them in ski boots, hiking shoes, daily shoes, everything. But if your feet are happy without them, it will save you some weight not to use them. I also need solid support for my arch and ankle; well, I have always needed it, because my packs usually weighed more than 40 pounds, and I have an ankle injury that predisposes my ankle to weakness under certain conditions. With the new ultralight approach, it appears the light pack does mean a low hiking shoe or new, high-tech trail-running shoe would be sufficient, even for my feet. I have spent many hours in such shoes on the trail, with packs that are less than 20 pounds and have had no problems. I just never put it into this context. Because part of this entire transition is the process of considering new options and giving them a try, I tested this theory. I took out my new pack filled with 30 pounds (a bridge pack with all my gear and a ton of flour to represent group gear and my food for a week). Bottom line: I found that for me, in very rugged terrain, my shoes do not provide enough support, especially on very steep, rugged downhill bushwhacks. But on trails, they were fine. So some of my trips will include the boots and some the shoes.

Some factors to consider here:

- ❁ If total pack weight is less than 20 pounds, will a lightweight hiking shoe or trail-running shoe suffice?

- ❁ You can easily install orthotics into any shoe, so you don't need a boot to use them.

- ❁ The lighter the weight on each foot, the less effort it takes to walk each step of the trek. Weight does matter.

- ❁ What makes your feet happy? Pick shoes/boots that fit well, that don't produce blisters, that support your arch and ankle as needed, fit with orthotics installed (if you need them), are comfortable and breathable, and that you like wearing.

- ❁ Don't forget to wear high-quality wicking socks that will help keep your feet dry and blister-free.

- ❁ Give yourself permission to have two sets of footwear: shoes for shorter, easier trips, and boots for longer, more difficult trips.

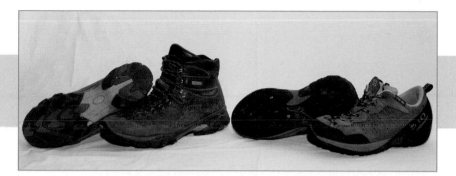

For each specific trip, pick the right kind of foot gear.

## Quick Tips

✓ Pick hiking shoes, running shoes, or boots that fit your feet well and are supportive for the needs of your arches and ankles.

✓ Use orthotic insoles to help reduce foot fatigue and align the bones of the foot and ankle.

✓ Lightest weight might not be the best fit for all trips. Choose the right footgear for each specific trip.

> *It always rains on tents. Rainstorms will travel thousands of miles, against prevailing winds for the opportunity to rain on a tent.*
>
> —DAVE BARRY

# The Shelter, Sleeping, and Lighting System

ALONG WITH THE WEIGHT of the pack itself, this system comprises the biggest reduction in weight between the conventional and ultralight approaches. Here is where the difference in mindset is most apparent. Let's begin with shelters.

In the late 1990s, we took a group of Boy Scouts to the Grand Canyon north-rim area of Deer Creek. This trip included a number of events that made it memorable, but the one that has to do with sheltering is of interest here. Our permit required us to camp just below the upper Deer Creek falls, in an area full of bushes. There were no trees nearby to hang food or trash to keep it from critters in the night, so we used the bushes, stringing a line across our cramped campsite above our sleeping bags. It was a lovely night, so we slept under the stars, four of us side by side in the only flat area not covered by bushes. In the middle of the night, I was awakened by a sickening complaint by my friend Rick, who apparently sat up in bed to go pee and found his bed covered in what felt like bloody goo. When it's completely dark and you are half asleep, blind, and silent in the middle of the night, placing your hand unexpectedly in such a puddle on your bed can invigorate the imagination and stimulate action! Upon investigation with headlamps, we discovered that a ringtail cat had walked the line holding our trash bags, and apparently dispersed the leftover pudding from the night before onto Rick's sleeping bag, along with a number of other tasty items. The definition of shelter took on a new meaning after that night.

## HOME AWAY FROM HOME

The conventional approach is to use a tent as the means to protect yourself from the elements. Most backpacking tents are double-walled tents comprised of a tent body and a rainfly, supported by shock-corded aluminum poles. Many of these are freestanding, which is very nice in many situations. At the other end of the spectrum, we find a tiny pad with a quilt on top, sleeping under the stars. There are, of course, many variations on this spectrum. Combined with the warmth gear (sleeping bag or quilt in combination with warm clothes), we can create many types of functional sleeping systems. Before examining these, let's consider what's important to you for three-season backpacking.

- Are you OK sleeping under the stars, with no other protection overhead?

- Do you need rain protection at night?

- Do you need bug protection at night?

- How much cushion do you need under you, between you and the hard ground? How much insulation is needed underneath you to keep you warm?

- Do you need padding under your legs and feet?

- Do you roll around at night or pretty much stay put once you fall asleep?

- Are you a side sleeper or a back sleeper? What kind of pad meets your needs the best?

- Do you get cold easily? Do you overheat easily?

- What is the coldest temperature you expect to endure with this sleep system?

- Do you prefer a quilt, sleeping bag, or combo of layering clothes and one of these?

- Where you like to backpack, how hard is it to stake out guy lines? Can you use stakes or tie to rocks, or do you require a freestanding shelter?

- What is required to make it easy for you to enter and exit the shelter, both in daylight and at night?

- Is your sleep system functional if your pack and clothes are totally wet from rain?

- If it's pouring, can you get into and out of your shelter without soaking what's inside the shelter? Can you change clothes inside your shelter?

From this list we can determine what kind of sleep/shelter system will best meet your needs and desires.

The ultralight backpacker values simplicity. The basic sleep system of many ultralighters is a simple piece of closed-cell foam, a quilt, and a tarp. Yet, for many conventional trekkers this would be extremely uncomfortable. My goal is to preserve comfort while minimizing weight. So we need to step into this mindset from the bridge perspective.

Today's tent technology is truly amazing! There are some really cool shelters out there. Some are freestanding; many are not. Some are built to withstand expedition blizzards, others are intended for three-season backpacking, and still others are uniquely ultralight. The more I searched, the more variety I found, and I discovered a number of unique tiny companies selling ultralight gear. Some had pretty high recommendations from their customers. None were sold at major retail stores.

I began my search by being clear about my requirements. For three-season backpacking, these were my tent decisions:

- ⚙ It would be OK if my tent were not freestanding.

- ⚙ The tent needed to weigh less than 2 pounds.

- ⚙ The tent needed to be a full-coverage tent—that is, bug protection as well as rain protection

- ⚙ It had to be easy to use, easy to enter/exit, easy to dress in, sleep, and so on.

- ⚙ It had to have at least a small vestibule to shelter my boots outside of the living space

This list ruled out all of the ultralight tarps as well as most, if not all, of the freestanding tents, the tarps not being full coverage and the freestanding tents being too heavy.

Once I listed my requirements, I went through a similar process with what worked for packs. I purchased some and tried them out, comparing them to each other, in this case for the following:

- ⚙ comfort

- ⚙ ease of setup

* general durability
* number of poles required
* number of stakes required
* size of overall footprint
* trekking-pole use versus dedicated tent poles
* weatherproofness
* weight

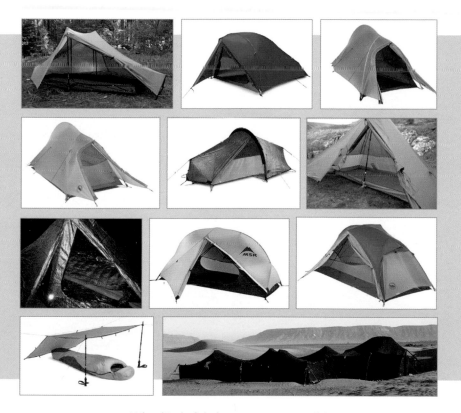

What kind of shelter meets your needs?

Three questions, in addition to all of the above, affected the final decision: Did I like it? Was it easy to use? Would it work for the kinds of backpacks I do, the places I like to go?

Some of the ultralight tents are made from traditional nylon (as are most conventional tents), which means they stretch after a while and you need to tighten the guy lines. These generally are cheaper to purchase and more readily available. Many of these ultralight tents seemed to be new inventions of the conventional non-freestanding tent, really a tarp plus some kind of inner tent, using a conventional style ground cloth under everything.

I found other tents made from Cuben Fiber, an ultralight, yet strong fabric that is waterproof and does not stretch. Cuben Fiber tents are much like traditional single-wall tents in that they often must deal with a lot of condensation. Some of the designs were very unique and creative in how to handle that moisture. (For example, Hexamid tents by Zpacks place the ground cloth inside the tent mesh so the moisture can run down the mesh outside of your ground cloth and onto the ground underneath.) The big thing about Cuben Fiber is that it is unbelievably light while still being strong (and, of course, more pricey).

The tent I liked best turned out to be one of the Cuben Fiber Hexamids, called the Hexamid Solo Plus (a bit larger than the Solo). It weighs 19.1 ounces without stakes, and only 23.3 ounces if I include a full suite of 10 stakes! All other tents I tested weighed more than this, did not meet the requirements listed above, or were not easy for me to use. The Hexamid uses only one trekking pole and takes only a few minutes to set up. Once up, it meets all of my requirements. It is

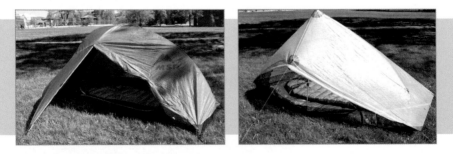

Conventional MSR Hubba or the ultralight Zpacks Hexamid Solo Plus?

## Quick Tips

✓ When choosing a shelter, be clear about your priorities and needs. What is important to you?

✓ Select the lightest shelter that will work (meet your needs) in most of the back-packs you do. Select the one that is best for what you usually do, yet will work in extreme cases, even if in those cases it will not be optimal.

✓ One kind of shelter may not be appropriate for all altitudes and seasons. You may need more than one.

roomy and comfortable and has plenty of room for gear inside the tent, along with vestibule coverage for boots outside the door. And since it does not stretch, once set up properly, I rarely need to adjust the tension in the lines. The only downside is that it requires 10 stakes, which means a bit of work setting it up. At first I balked at this, thinking that would be a showstopper. However, after setting it up a few times and then taking it on a number of treks, I found it to be a nonissue. And I have some extra cord to wrap rocks appropriately when I cannot pound stakes into the ground, although so far I have never had to use that cord. I also installed tiny ultralight cord tensioners on the tent-stake lines, allowing very easy adjustment of tautness. These don't come with the tent but are an ease-of-use item worth the tiny extra weight.

Several other tents might have worked OK, but simply were not as light. So in the end, usability and weight drove the decision. (For testing, as with packs, I purchased tents, carefully tested them, and then returned all but one of them.)

My conventional packing method for the shelter and sleeping system has been to break the tent into packages, tent body in one stuff sack, the fly in another, the poles in their own sack, and the stakes in theirs. The sleeping bag and liner go together in their sack along with sleeping clothes, and the pad is packed into a stuff sack alone. This approach makes it easy to pack and keeps my gear orderly. It requires six stuff sacks.

When using ultralight gear, however, life gets simpler. My ultralight tent is such a small package that it does not need to be broken up. In addition, the pad is so small it goes into the sleeping bag stuff sack rather than being a significant packing item in and of itself. This sack also contains the few extra clothes I bring: socks, skivvies, and a sleeping shirt. The new way of packing requires only two stuff sacks for the entire Shelter, Sleeping, and Lighting System.

## TO SLEEP, PERCHANCE TO DREAM

Comfort is king when it comes to sleeping systems. So the driving force for decisions on sleeping bags and pads comes down to two things:

- ⚙ How warm do you sleep? Are you a hot sleeper? Do you get cold easily? These drive the temperature rating of the sleeping bag or quilt.

- ⚙ How much cushion do you need (as well as how much insulation underneath you)? The pad decision determines how well you sleep almost as much as the warmth of the bag. They must work together.

Sleeping bags or quilts made from high-quality down are the obvious choices for ultralight backpacking due to the amazing characteristics of such down (for a given warmth, it compresses better than anything else, it is usually much lighter in weight, and it can be expected to outlast synthetic equivalents).

Down is rated by its insulation capabilities through what's known as its "fill factor." A single ounce of a specific quality of down is placed into a graduated cylinder under a known pressure. The down fluffs up inside the cylinder and the height to which the down rises is noted. If the down fills 500 cubic inches of space, it is called "500 fill down." If it fills 800, it is "800 fill." The finer the feathers, the more the feathers fill with air, so the higher the quality, the higher the fill factor. For sleeping bags, 800 fill and above are considered very high quality; 900 fill and above is considered extremely high quality. The higher the fill factor, the warmer and more compressible it will be for a given weight—and, of course, the more expensive it will be. (By the way, you can get the same warmth out of a lower-quality down. It will just take more of the down to do it, which means the sleeping bag will be heavier and less compressible.)

The counter consideration to choosing a down sleeping bag is whether or not you plan to spend much time in humid or seriously rainy conditions, in which case the down might absorb moisture and thereby lose its insulating capabilities. Down is worthless when it becomes wet, where synthetic insulation will still insulate when wet. But synthetics at the time of this writing are still heavier and less compressible than down for a given warmth rating. Still, if all of your trips are in the northwestern or southeastern US, it may be well worth the extra ounces to have a bag that still works in high humidity. In that case you also now have the option to choose products made with hydrophobic (water-repellent) down. These new bags (and jackets) are not as compressible as natural down, not quite as light in weight, but usually are better than synthetic counterparts. So as technology advances, so do our options.

European Norm Testing is a standardized rating system for the warmth of sleeping bags. It came out a few years ago and levels the playing field (now we can compare bags from very different vendors and insulations on an equal basis). EN testing includes placing a copper mannequin into the bag and then putting that into a climate chamber to do tests. The result is a consistent set of measurements for us to compare. The ratings include the temperature at which a "standard

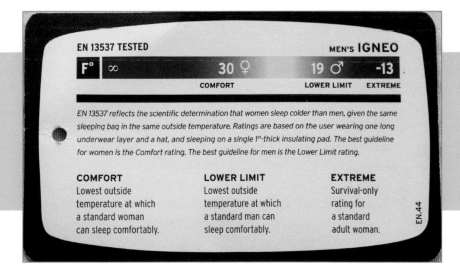

European Norm Testing Tag for Sleeping Bags

woman" would be comfortable, the temperature at which a "standard man" would be comfortable, and the temperature at which a "standard woman" can stay alive in this sleeping bag. *Standard* means that you are not a cold sleeper, nor a hot sleeper. These tests assume there is at least one inch of insulation beneath the bag, and that the person inside is wearing a light base layer top and bottom.

I usually add 10 degrees to the bag's rating for cold sleepers and subtract 5 degrees from the bag's rating for hot sleepers. This gives a pretty clear understanding of how well this bag will perform for most people. Don't forget that these ratings do not take into account wind, rain, humidity, personal eating habits, the day's exercise, and so on.

The purpose of your bed is to provide a good night's sleep. If you get cold easily, a quilt is probably not the best choice, because it does not keep out the cold from underneath you. So a sleeping bag is the choice for you. On the other hand, if you are a hot sleeper, a quilt will save you weight while providing a lovely down comforter to keep you warm. There are some sleeping bags today that have no insulation on the bottom, but instead they have a sleeve for your pad. These bags expect you to save weight through this mechanism, and they expect that you will buy into their "system" of doing things. It works well for those who like air mattresses or for those who worry about slipping off the pad. In my opinion this is not a good system for cold sleepers, but it might help to save some weight for warmer sleepers who want a full sleeping bag rather than a quilt.

Choose a quilt or bag that is rated to the coldest conditions you will regularly encounter. Don't buy for the one time in 10 years that you might do a winter trip. Buy for the everyday trips you take each year.

For my ultralight sleeping system, I chose a conventional sleeping bag rather than a quilt, a 20-degree down bag that weighs 26.6 ounces. This saved me only 0.1 ounce in weight but gained 10 degrees of warmth from my previous 30-degree, 26.7-ounce bag.

As for pads, for conventional trekking in the past, I have used a short (47- x 20-inch) 1.5-inch-thick self-inflating pad that weighs 16 ounces. In conjunction with this, I used my empty pack to provide a pad for my feet, and I have a small synthetic pillow to complete the package. To transition into ultralight gear, I chose to retain 1.5 inches of cush, but am now using a minimalist frame-style pad that is only 18 inches wide by 40 inches long, and it fits inside the sleeping bag. It is called the Klymit Inertia X-Lite and weighs only 7.3 ounces. Furthermore, I chose to bring an ultralight air pillow that weighs 1.4 ounces to support my neck.

This bag and pad in combination with my insulated pants and down jacket enable me to handle almost three seasons of high altitude or deep canyon camping, at a significant weight savings. Note that I mention my insulated pants here. Since my pad now does not provide insulation under my legs, and the new bridge pack has little in that regard as well (which is under my calves and feet), under colder conditions it is necessary for me to wear the insulated pants inside the sleeping bag as part of my pad-provided insulation. If my pack is wet from the day's activities, I can substitute my hiking pants folded roughly into a square pad as the insulation under my feet. In this case I also use a stuff sack filled with gear (such as gloves, hats, and clothes) under my knees. This system works well if the ground is warm (as in summer and fall); for high-altitude spring (or winter) trips, however, I need more insulation under my sleeping bag. The lightest pad that

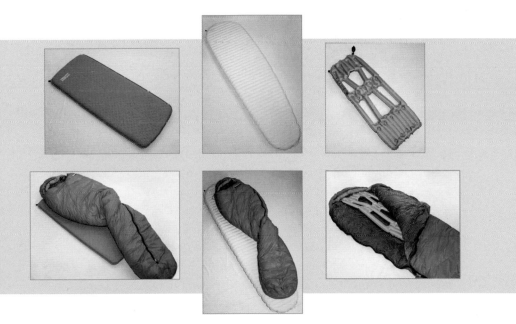

Pad design affects weight, cushion, and insulation.

## *Quick Tips*

 Don't select a sleeping bag because you need a sleeping bag. Instead, design your sleeping system as an entity, and then purchase the appropriate parts (bag or quilt, pad, insulated clothes, etc.).

✓ The sleeping bag and pad work together to provide insulation under and over you. They provide no warmth. What you eat and how you exercise, in combination with your metabolism, create the heat that keeps you warm. Be sure to include your diet and nutrition in the equation when you consider how to stay warm at night.

✓ European Norm Testing gives us the most reliable warmth ratings to compare sleeping bags. Be sure to take into account whether you get cold easily or are a hot sleeper, and appropriately modify the ratings.

works for me as a "back sleeper" is the Thermarest NeoAir XLite in size large. This was the lightest back-sleeper-supportive pad I could find at the time (summer 2013). It does impact my weight—I'm back to 16 ounces—but the good night's sleep is worth it. Another gear feature used only when needed for specific trips.

## LET THERE BE LIGHT

The "lighting" part of this system is my headlamp, which conventionally lives in with my repair kit in the top pocket of the pack, always ready if needed, with a spare in my first-aid kit. Under the new ultralight approach, the light is still packed in with the repair items, but weighs less. The spare headlamp stays home, replaced by one extra battery. (Unless the trip is an expedition, in which case I take the spare light and extra batteries. By the way, I always use commercially available lithium batteries that are much lighter to carry; they work better in cold weather and last longer than alkaline or rechargeable batteries.) Headlamps give the ability to function hands-free while still having light. There are many variations available, all varying in weight and features. Many are rated in brightness using "lumens" as the relative amount of light they produce.

If you only use it to read, then a light that produces 35 lumens is probably OK. If you are hiking at night, you probably want more light, something in the range of 70–130 lumens. If you are doing search-and-rescue work, you might want a really powerful light in the range of 200 lumens of light. So what you choose must be based on how you plan to use it. My conventional choice was a Black Diamond Spot, an older version rated at 90 lumens max, with a continuous dimmer; a mid-range setting, also dimmable; the option to use red light to save night vision; and a lockout mechanism so it won't accidentally turn on in my pack. It weighs 3.1 ounces and uses three AAA batteries. My new replacement headlamp produces 97 lumens at its max, with a mid setting of 47 lumens and a low setting of 3 lumens. It weighs less than 1 ounce and uses only one AA battery. (I take the battery out of the unit when hiking and install it as evening approaches. This ensures it won't accidentally turn on in my pack.)

As you compare headlamps, check out their ability to handle weather via their waterproofness. Most carry an IP (Ingress Protection) Code rating such as "IPX-4," "IPX-7," or "IPX-8." The four means it can handle rain or snow or splashing, but cannot be submerged and still work. The eight means the light can be dropped into a meter or two of water and when removed from the water it will still work. The IP Code is an industry standard that rates the durability of products. It includes many aspects, but the one we are interested in is the one related to ingress of water. The range is from one to eight, and covers affects of dripping water through spraying water through total immersion. The X in this case has to do with dust ingress and can be assumed to be almost as high as the water rating, with the X indicating that no claim to dust protection is noted.

In addition to the original questions listed at the beginning of this section, for lighting we also need to ask:

- How do you plan to use light? Is a headlamp appropriate (hands-free operation)? Is it sufficient? Do you need a lantern or flashlight?

- Will you need to hike at night when it is very dark? If so, are you just hiking, or will you be searching?

- Will you need to set up camp in the dark?

&#9881; Do you need to preserve night vision while having a light on? (This requires a red light.)

&#9881; How waterproof do you need the headlamp to be?

&#9881; Do you need a lantern or candle for ambient light (such as in a snow shelter)?

These questions help determine how bright your light should be and what style is most appropriate for your uses.

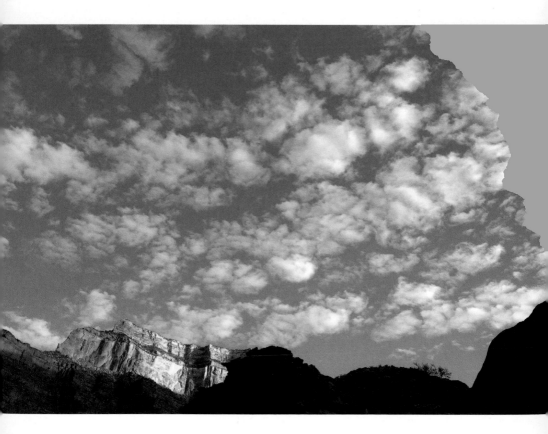

*Nothing is more imminent than the impossible ... what we must always foresee is the unforeseen.*

—VICTOR HUGO

# The Three Smaller Systems:
## Navigation System; First-Aid, Repair, and Personal-Hygiene System; Communication System

These are important systems in all kinds of backpacking, but their contents might change from conventional to ultralight use. It depends on the kinds of trips you are taking as to how complete these systems need to be. For example, if you are leading treks where you need to navigate without trails, bushwhacking through rugged terrain, your navigation and first-aid systems may need to be more thorough and involved than if you are hiking on known trails with few obstacles while leading experienced trekkers. This is true for both conventional and ultralight arrangements.

### AM I LOST?

On one trip about 15 years ago, we were descending into Young's Canyon in Utah, on a rough but discernible trail, when we encountered two men hiking up out of the canyon. Upon greeting them, we discovered they were extremely upset. It became apparent that after hiking all the way to the river, they had found no US Forest Service sign at the river telling them which way was upstream and which way was downstream! So they had no choice but to retreat toward whence they came. We were flabbergasted, amused, and actually delighted that they were going home, so we would not have to rescue them! Wow. Something about common sense comes to mind . . . . This, of course, applies to both conventional and ultralight backpacking.

Navigation must always include a map and compass. The compass can be much simpler and smaller for ultralight trips, especially if trekking on well-traveled trails. Maps can be trimmed if you want to be really ultralight, allowing you to take only the part(s) of the map you need. All backpackers should know how to use a map and compass.

GPS units augment but do not replace a map and compass. Conventional backpackers often use handheld field GPS units to help in navigation, and these units offer many fun features. Ultralight trekkers often either do not use GPS units or wear a lighter-weight GPS watch to accomplish what is necessary. This last word is key: Ultralight means only take what is necessary. (And, of course, GPS units are not worth their weight if you do not know how to set them up, calibrate the components that need it, and use the features.)

## FIRST-AID, CONTINGENCY, AND REPAIR KITS

My conventional first-aid kit, which I've carried for years now, weighs a little more than 2 pounds! My repair kit with extra batteries and an emergency bivvy is another pound. In my defense, I have been leading treks into rugged and remote areas of the Grand Canyon for more than 20 years. Over that span, I have had to use my SAM splint three times on broken ankles in the backcountry. I've also seen someone slide down slickrock resulting in really bad road rash for which a large first-aid kit was needed to treat the wounds. After this experience, and then

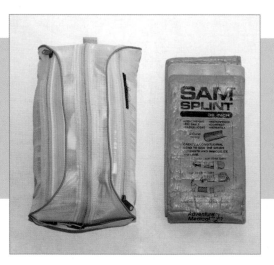

First-Aid Kit

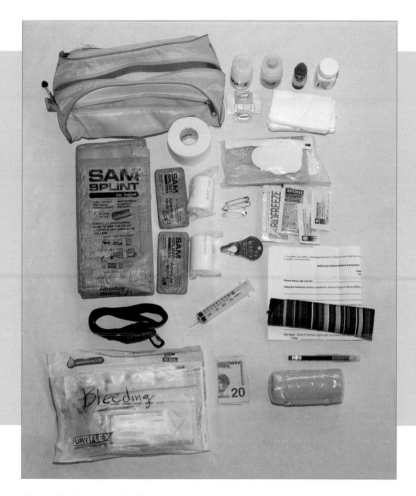

First-Aid Kit (Expanded View)

taking the NOLS (National Outdoor Leadership School) 16-hour Wilderness First Aid course, my kit grew even bigger. (Full disclosure: Since then I've never used even a Band-Aid from it!)

The ultralight approach to first-aid and repair supplies is simple. Just take what you might need for yourself for a couple of days. It's enough. If you need more, you'll improvise. If you go into really rough terrain, take a SAM splint along. SAMs are pretty light and can also be used as part of some other system, for example, as a cozy around a freeze-dried meal when "cooking." (If you are a guide or leader of trips into rough terrain, someone in the group should have a more complete first-aid kit, or the group can organize such that, when combined, all of their first-aid supplies add up to a complete kit.) I tried very hard to apply this approach, eliminating everything I could. In the end, I found that I could only lighten my first-aid kit a bit, because I still feel the need to handle any serious situation in the backcountry, especially as the leader of treks. So I'm still carrying 24.2 ounces of first-aid gear (that includes a SAM splint).

The place we can save a good deal of weight is in the knife/multitool arena. Many ultralighters only take a simple one-sided razor blade as their knife. You can easily make a protective case for it out of cardboard and some tape. Take two if you need a backup. They are unbelievably light and small to pack.

I have often carried two knives in my pack, one in the first-aid kit and one in the repair kit, one backing up the other. And, in the last two decades, I don't think I've used either one on a backpacking trip. I carry a tiny pair of scissors in my first-aid kit, and that's all I've ever needed. Careful planning ahead of trips

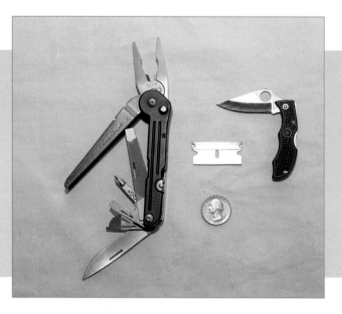

How much of a cutting tool do you need?

often eliminates the need for a knife. I know that this is a religious issue for some folks who use knives for everything. But if you really are honest about what is actually necessary, you may find this is an area where you can save weight. Yet, a knife is a far better tool for survival than a razor blade, especially in winter. I was recently given a tiny Spyderco knife, quite small, very well made, and weighing 0.5 ounce. Since it is big enough to actually carve with, it has become a bridge for me to ensure survival, replacing one of my razor blades (which were replacing the knives), the other razor blade being a backup for the Spyderco. You must decide for each trip what is appropriate to take, considering the odds that you will need to spend a night or two surviving off the land. In the next section there are more thoughts on contingency planning.

For winter trips, I can see the need for a really hefty Leatherman kind of multiuse tool, specifically for ski and snowshoe binding repair. And I can see the use of pliers to help sew a heavy backpack or boot together if necessary. However, we're not using heavy backpacks or boots in our three-season ultralight setup, so the floss we bring for sewing can easily be hand-sewn into the light pack material of our ultralight gear. Thus, for some trips we can lighten up by leaving both the knife and the tool at home.

Some questions you might want to consider as you design your first-aid and repair kits:

- Are you responsible for only your own injuries, or do you need to be able to help others?

- Is your kit expected to be part of a larger group kit composed of specific items to support the group?

- What's the worst situation or accident you need to be prepared to handle, realistically? Does this situation require specific gear or just knowledge?

- What's the minimum collection of supplies that will enable you to handle what you need to handle?

- When was the last time you took any kind of first-aid course? Have you taken a NOLS Wilderness First Aid course or equivalent (these are really good)? Do you need a refresher?

⚙     Can you get double or triple use from any of these items; can they be used to meet other backpacking needs?

⚙     How accessible does your gear need to be? Can you break it into smaller pieces to be more effective? (For example, blister gear might need easy access, where other items can be packed elsewhere.)

⚙     What do you expect to be repairing? What is the minimum you need to accomplish those repairs?

## Quick Tips

✓     First-aid and repair gear should be considered part of your contingency planning. Think carefully about what you really need to have along.

✓     Do you need to take into account the need for overnight survival (or longer perhaps)? If so, your repair and first-aid kits might need to include different items.

✓     SAM splints come in several sizes. I carry one that can be used for arms, legs, necks, and so on, as well as a couple of finger-size ones. The longer and more remote the trek, the higher the probability that you might need to use one of these. Watch SAM training videos—they are short and well made.

## PERSONAL HYGIENE IN THE BACKCOUNTRY

On one trip to the Canyonlands with Boy Scouts, we were approaching our campsite area after a long, hot hike to camp. As we arrived at the camping area, one boy dropped his pack, ditched his shirt, and began rolling and frolicking in the beach-like sand of the small hill next to camp. Soon he was caked in sand stuck to his sweaty body. We stood there, appalled and shocked by this behavior, unable to even think of what to say. So we decided to let him be and set up camp. In the end, his approach might have been even better than our own in some respects, although perhaps not as healthy. He quickly soaked up the sticky sweat on his body into the sand, and then, of course, the sand dried on his body. When he brushed it off, he was then dry and cooler than he had been before (and maybe even cleaner, but nobody knows). The down side was that bugs that were in the sand bit him, giving him a number of itchy welts as a result. So far, we have not repeated his unique approach to hygiene.

Everyone gets dirty backpacking, but staying healthy for more than an overnight requires a daily hygiene routine that is carefully planned, well established, religiously followed, and easy to do. It often is just bathing or washing, having healthy bowel movements daily, brushing teeth, and ensuring that hands are clean before meals. These principles apply to all backpacking styles and, of course, vary according to altitude, weather, and location. Of most interest here is how to do this well, efficiently, and in as lightweight a manner as possible.

Long ago I learned that a tiny towel that absorbs many times its weight in water was a wonderful thing in the backcountry. It can be used as a washcloth as well as a towel, and depending on the particular fabric, will continue to be absorbent enough to dry skin even when it is wet from washing. There are many kinds available today, but the smallest or next-to-smallest ones are big enough to do the job yet tiny to pack, weigh very little, and often absorb as much as eight times their weight in water. So leave the large towel, washcloth, and bathrobe at home! In addition, soap is often bad for the environment, even the biodegradable kind, in backcountry conditions. For the daily bath, a brisk skinny dip into a running mountain stream or pool will do wonders. Then a bit of sanitizing gel on your hands and face, and voilà, you are clean. So far, that means we only have to carry a tiny towel and a tiny plastic bottle of sanitizer. Add to this your toothbrush (cut in half to save weight) and a small plastic bottle partially filled with tooth powder. This is extremely lightweight and lasts a long time.

These are the basics, but what else might we take with us related to hygiene? I often bring a small bottle or tube of lotion, which can be used for sunburn and dry skin, as well as for first aid when necessary. In addition, some people bring specific medicines that are of a personal nature for themselves or possibly for others, medications not normally in their first-aid gear but that apply to a particular trip or circumstance: allergy-reaction medications, asthma inhalers, cold-sore medications, ear-infection drops, EpiPens, and so on. Repackaging these can be tricky but might help lighten them. Use common sense here.

Trip leaders should bring extra hand sanitizer and medicines just in case. (By the way, I have some friends who don't bring sanitizer; they just never touch their food with their hands. This is their way of ensuring health in the backcountry.)

For most backpacking meals, with freeze-dried dinners or the like, the only dishes that get dirty are my spoon and possibly my cup. And for these, after I've cleaned them well with my tongue and a hot cup of tea; I use a tiny bit of boiling water to rinse them after each meal. If cooking complex meals, soap can be important, especially when the pots get oily or greasy such that sand-scrubbing in a stream followed by boiling water is not enough. In these cases, I bring biodegradable soap, otherwise I leave it at home. For breakfasts I have my nuts and oats, and so on, in a sandwich-size baggie. Sometimes I put that baggie into my cup and fold the top outward to open the bag and overlap the lip of the cup. Then I pour some hot water in and have breakfast. Other times I just pour directly into the baggie while it is resting on a rock or solid surface. This way I free up the cup so I can have my tea at the same time. The baggie approach means I have no cleanup afterward except my spoon, and the hot tea takes care of that easily.

## THREE-SEASON CONTINGENCY PLANNING

Some thoughts on contingency preparedness:

Obviously, we cannot take everything needed to handle all possible situations that might occur in the backcountry. But we can be prepared to handle some reasonable set of possibilities. One approach to this is to have a selection of generic tools available that cover a number of situations. These can be part of, rather than in addition to, what you have in your first-aid and repair kits. (Also see "Winter Contingency Planning," page 114.)

The list that follows is a trimmed-down version of what I've used for conventional treks for many years. Reconsidering this through the viewpoint of ultralight thinking enabled me to save some weight and still be prepared. Some example contingency tools are listed here (you should modify this list as appropriate for each trip and your preferences).

- athletic tape
- blood-clot bandage to stop serious bleeding
- chlorine dioxide tablets or drops
- contingency food (jerky or other high-protein, long-lasting, lightweight food)
- curved sewing needle
- duct tape

- one-eighth-inch nylon cord, perhaps 30–50 feet

- emergency reflective bivvy

- extra battery for headlamp

- extra straps, with easy to clip buckles

- fine-point permanent marker (such as Sharpie)

- floss to use as thread or survival trap or string

- one-sided razor blade in cardboard carrying case (and/or multiuse tool or knife in specific cases)

- pencil and paper

- reading glasses (if needed)

- SAM splint

- small Bic lighter

- some 0000-grade (very fine) steel wool (to be used in conjunction with extra battery to start a fire)

## COMMUNICATION GEAR

One quick note on communication gear:

Sometimes communication gear is paramount. Other kinds of trips don't need it. You need to decide for each trip if it warrants carrying the extra weight. In "Assessing and Managing Risk" (page 130), I detail a Grand Canyon trip to Nankoweep in which we had serious issues to deal with. We were able to save a participant's life, salvage the trip, keep everyone else safe even with additional injuries, and deal calmly with this unexpected emergency, in part because we had radios. The big factor here was that we had a larger group of hikers who tended to spread out on the trail. If we had been only three or four, the dynamic would have been much different.

Also, if we had only had ultralight packs, the impact would have been so very much less. As it was, two of us each carried more than 60 pounds with our own gear and half of the injured person's. If we had been using ultralight gear, our weight might have increased from 20 to 30 pounds instead of 40 to 60. A much different problem!

*Sir, respect your dinner: idolize it, enjoy it properly. You will be many hours in the week, many weeks in the year, and many years in your life happier if you do.*

—WILLIAM MAKEPEACE THACKERAY

# The Fire and Nutrition Systems

TOGETHER WITH THE PACK itself and the Sleeping and Shelter System, the Fire and Nutrition Systems are the heaviest items we have to carry. Food and water are always the heaviest items we have along unless the trip is extremely short, or in some cases if water is accessible en route enough to allow us to carry minimal hydration. So how we plan our meals and hydration will impact the overall effort required for the trip. The items included in this arena are the following:

- cooking pot(s) to match the stove in size and the kind of cooking to be done
- food, snacks, all nutritional items
- overnight food storage
- stove(s) and appropriate fuel
- water purification/filtration system and hydration container(s)—bottles, bladders, in-camp containers

This is an important area for trip planning, as exemplified by this story from one of my earliest Backpacking Basics classes. A man took my class and then went on a four-day backpacking trip. He came back complaining that it was a horrible experience and wanted me to help him figure out what he did wrong. He explained that he was coughing up blood, felt very weak, had to force himself to hike 8 miles with a light day pack on his layover day, and then came home feeling terrible. We weighed his pack and gear, we checked his list of what he took, and he did it all pretty well, with one exception. He had decided that he would take only two Clif bars as his nutrition so he could lose some weight. His only food for four days was two energy bars!

When you go backpacking, your body requires MORE nutrition than usual, not less. This is NOT the time to try to lose some weight. Rather, it is a time to eat extra calories to give you the energy you need to carry a pack and hike many miles with a smile on your face. This is far more important if your pack is a conventional weight, the terrain is rough, and the mileage is high. We will first consider the fire system, then food, then hydration.

## THE STOVE AND ITS POT

The Fire System includes not only some means of creating a fire in an emergency, but also your cook stove, fuel, and pots. For emergency fire planning, I usually just take a snack-size zip-top baggie with some 0000-grade steel wool in it. If ever needed, I hold the ends of the steel wool to the ends of a spare battery, and voilà! Be careful—the steel wool will turn gold and possibly white as it heats up and will burn you if you are not careful in how you hold it to the battery. This hot element is then just right for igniting tiny kindling. I sometimes also take some waterproof matches to cover emergencies if I expect to be in really wet conditions.

As experienced conventional backpackers will attest, the stove and pot choices are closely related to the Nutrition System, because which stove and pots you need are directly influenced by the kind of meals you plan to prepare. So the choice must be made for each trip depending on:

- how many people are being fed,
- the number of stoves and pots available,
- water availability near campsites,
- the duration of the trip, and
- what meals are being served.

Consider the following chart, showing the relationship of stove and pot type to the kinds of food being prepared:

| KIND OF MEALS COOKED | STOVE AND POT(S) REQUIRED |
|---|---|
| Just boiling water (freeze-dried or home-dried meals). | Efficient, hot stove; any pot to hold the water. It's nice to have larger pots for larger groups of people; small pots are fine for few people. |
| Actually cooking meals like pasta, stews, and so on. | Stove must simmer well; pot must be big enough for what's being cooked. Nonstick is a plus. |
| Frying fish, cooking meats or whole grains, sautéing, gourmet meals, and so on. | Stove must simmer well; pot must be big enough. Lid or frying pan must be available with handle. |

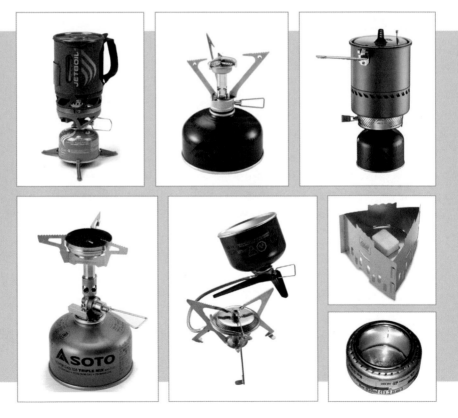

Some Lighter-Weight Stove Options

## Quick Tips

✓ The stove and pot are a team that must work together according to the kinds of cooking and meals you plan on each trip. Pick the combination that works best for each specific trip.

✓ Wind and rain can play havoc with stoves and meal preparation if not properly planned for. The happiness of your campers may depend on how well you can cook in adverse conditions. A well-thought-out choice of stove and pot may save your trip.

✓ Weight may not be the most important factor when choosing a stove. Bridging in this arena can mean less frustration and more happiness on a trip. This is an area where minimizing hassle may override extra weight.

For long trips, having backup stoves is imperative. I usually take one stove for every three to four people. But the minimum number for any trip is two stoves. It is very helpful if the fuel can be shared among the stoves taken. Hence, take stoves that share the same type of fuel; that is, all canister stoves or all liquid-fuel stoves or all alcohol-burning, and so on. In addition, if warranted, be sure to take stoves that can handle windy conditions, or bring extra fuel for the inefficiency in flame control under such conditions. Some stoves whose vendors tout that they are windproof are not. Others, like the MSR Reactor, are. So you need to test the stove you plan to use to be sure it performs in wind to your satisfaction. Usually, stoves that allow a wind screen (canister stoves that separate the canister from the burner, or liquid-fuel stoves) will be sufficient.

How might the conventional backpacker change meal and stove planning to accommodate lighter gear choices? Again, the bridge concept plays a role. My experience has shown that the lightest, smallest stoves are great for some trips and horrible on others, usually depending on the weather (wind and rain or snow). For rough weather conditions, my MSR Windpro II outshines all of its lighter brothers because it is almost impervious to wind. It weighs 6 ounces, where my Soto Windmaster weighs less than 3 ounces but does not do as well in windy conditions. So for me, the lack of frustration from having a stove that works well in bad weather is more than worth the extra 3 ounces. As with other considerations, choose the right stove for each trip, rather than just one stove for all trips. Winter trips also require careful thought in this regard. (See "Winter Considerations," page 95, for more ideas.) For pots, in addition to the kind of food being cooked, it depends on how many people per stove are being served. If just boiling water, a 1-liter teapot works fantastically for one or two people with a tiny stove, allowing a very light and efficient system. However, for larger groups its nice to have larger pots, hence possibly different stoves. For Grand Canyon treks with larger groups, I usually take the larger Windpro II with a larger pot to handle both the wind and the ability to boil more water per potful. This is part of the "group gear" and is, of course, a trade-off of weight for better group support.

Some thoughts on stove and pot choices:

⚙ Specifically "ultralight" stove choices include only stoves that weigh less than a few ounces (and might not be limited to):

◇ *commercial alcohol stoves*

◇ *Esbit solid-fuel stoves*

◇ *homemade Coke-can alcohol stoves*

◇ *lightweight isobutene propane canister stoves*

⚙ Determining factors in choice of stove:

◇ *availability of fuel*

◇ *commonness of the stove (how easy is it to share fuel with others)*

◇ *cooking time based on how hot a flame the stove produces*

◇ *ease of use*

◇ *fuel efficiency*

◇ *fuel weight*

◇ *size of the pots the stove can support*

◇ *size of the stove*

◇ *weather conditions and altitudes in which the stove can still operate well*

◇ *weight of the stove*

- Determining factors in choice of pot(s):

    - *ease of use, ease of cleaning (nonstick?)*

    - *pot size in relation to the stove that is chosen*

    - *presence of handles, whether they're insulated, whether a potholder is needed*

    - *shape and size of pot with regard to what can be packed inside it (stove, cup, fuel canister, etc.)*

    - *size of pot in liters of liquid it can hold*

    - *types of food the pot can cook (water only, pasta and soups, frying)*

    - *versatility of pot—can it work on other stoves or only a specific stove?*

    - *weight of the pot*

    - *whether a lid is included or not*

- Solo backpacking allows freedom to choose the smallest, lightest options

- Group treks may require stoves and pots that are larger and heavier.

- Windy conditions can play havoc with many stoves and ruin many a meal. Appropriate choice of stove ahead of time can minimize frustration and might even save a trip.

- Piezoelectric stove igniters do not always work; often in colder temperatures they fail to produce a spark. So, a butane lighter is a good thing to have along.

- Some trips are designed around meals that are gourmet, cooked in the wild, creative, and fun. These usually require different stoves and pots from those used in fast-tracking or more usual backpacking trips, in which meals are freeze-dried or no-cook in order to minimize meal-preparation effort and fuel use.

- A 16- to 20-fluid-ounce titanium pot can double as the cooking pot and as a bowl or cup. Even for conventional trips I usually only take one cup for both bowl and cup use. The downside is that you can't have your tea and your soup simultaneously in separate containers.

- A 1-liter titanium or aluminum teapot works well for boiling water and works well on small stoves. Appropriate for one to four people using one stove. This does not support simmering soups or stews or pasta.

&#9673;   Superefficient stove/pot combo systems (like the Jetboil or MSR Reactor) can be wonderful, especially for winter use if the stove includes a regulator and a large enough pot for melting snow. Be careful that what you choose is appropriate for the kind of cooking you desire (some of these stoves do not simmer as well as other stove types, and some are wind-affected). They may or may not be lighter than some other stove/pot combinations (such as any tiny canister stove and a lightweight pot). They are often not as versatile as other stove systems, especially for larger groups. (See "Winter Considerations," page 95, for more discussion of these stoves.)

## FOOD IS NOT JUST FOOD

When we were training Boy Scouts to be prepared for longer backpacks, we instituted an annual event that proved to be very valuable. This was an overnight backpack for the boys that had an easy side-access for parents to visit our campsite. The boys (and we) would backpack 3 miles in to a special campsite, spend the night there, and then on Sunday morning, Mother's Day, the parents would hike a half mile into our camp to have the boys cook breakfast for them. We gave the boys complete freedom as to what and how to cook for this breakfast, which proved quite innovative and informative. Some of the things they came up with were extremely colorful and very creative (and often inedible). Others were very clever and practical. This is where we discovered that eggs could be taken to camp in a plastic bag, water boiled, the bag inserted into the boiling water, and voilà, scrambled eggs for breakfast with no cleanup mess. This could then become a breakfast burrito or other creative gift for your mom. We also learned that Tang, bacon, and Jell-O do not mix together quite as well as one might hope.

The proper food in the backcountry can determine the success or failure of your trip, along with how fun or horrible it is. Good nutrition is central to having the energy and health you need to handle the rigors that backcountry living demands. Careful food planning can minimize weight while ensuring healthy meals and snacks. This area requires some time to set up ahead of the trek, but is well worth the time spent up front at home. Here are my rules for meals based on preparing specific menus rather than carrying bulk foods as a pantry (as one might do for months in the backcountry):

⚙  Breakfast must be able to be accomplished only by boiling water so there will be no cleanup mess and breaking camp can be simplified. (Home-made "cereal" in a zip-top sandwich baggie works well, usually made from oats, nuts, dried fruits, and anything else you like. Just pour in hot water, have a lovely breakfast, and then place the baggie into your trash bag. No cleanup necessary, except the spoon.)

⚙  Lunches are no-cook. We never bring out the stoves for lunch or snacks (with the exception of some winter treks).

⚙  Dinners are fun to share. Plan them so everyone can eat at the same time and share the same basic kinds of foods (freeze-dried or cooked from scratch), stoves and pots, and so on. This makes the trip more fun and more relaxing, and provides the means for contingency. (If everyone is using the same kind of fuel and cooking the same style of meal, when a stove fails, the meal being prepared on the failed stove can easily be completed on another stove in the group.)

⚙  Dinners can be simple to prepare, but do not have to be boring. Don't forget soups and desserts. These not only add calories and great taste, but also can add important hydration, as well as creativity.

⚙  Trail snacks are as important as meals. Keeping your blood sugar and elec-trolytes balanced throughout the day helps give energy and support health. Plan snacks when you are planning meals. Bring only snacks that give great nutritional benefits. Don't just bring candy. Measure them out carefully so as not to carry unnecessary weight.

⚙  If you want some pizzazz, consider using two pots to create a double boiler. This can offer the opportunity to bake luscious things with little bother (like homemade cheesecake in the wild). If you plan ahead, life can indeed be very good. (Put small sticks in the bottom of the larger pot, pour in water, bring to boil, and then put in the smaller pot containing the goodies. Put lids on both, and "bake" away!)

⚙  No matter how hard I try to minimize weight, it usually ends up that I need between 1.25 and 1.5 pounds of food per day, more on some trips, especially in winter. That includes three meals, trail snacks, and any in-camp snacks, all food items consumed.

- Hydration is nutrition, especially in desert areas, high altitude (above 10,000 feet), and steep or difficult terrain. Don't forget to hydrate between arriving at camp and bedtime, and between waking and hitting the trail. I recommend a liter or more at each of these liminal times, especially in the desert.

- Repackaging food has always been a good idea, but becomes obligatory in the ultralight world. Pack food items logically and with minimal packaging for maximum ease of use with minimum weight. Organize food items according to when they will be used. Pack all items for each specific meal together.

- I take a 20-liter Ultrasil nylon dry bag as my "bear bag" to hang my food up at night. It weighs very little and provides a couple of nice features, namely, (1) it is waterproof so my food stays dry in storms, and (2) the waterproofness keeps in smells much better than regular stuff sacks, so critters are not as attracted to my food. It also clips nicely onto a rope loop or branch, so I don't need carabiners or other means to hang the bag. If where you are going requires a bear canister for food storage, use it instead of this dry bag.

- I carry smelly items like beef jerky and my premixed breakfast baggies in a Loksak Opsak odor-proof zip-top bag. These really work well to keep odors from attracting unwanted friends who want to eat your food, and they are light enough to be worth the effort.

- Never rush a meal. One of the main reasons I go into the backcountry is to enjoy being there. Meals provide an opportunity to relax and revel in wilderness surroundings. With proper planning, even meals in storms can be fun rather than stressful.

- Always bring some extra food as contingency in case you need to spend an unexpected night on the trail.

To get the most nutrition in terms of calories and energy per ounce of food, use foods high in carbs with a good balance of protein and fat, preferably real food with lots of trace minerals and vitamins, and so on. Nuts and nut butters are good trail snacks. Dinners and breakfasts should be lightweight and easy to fix. To be most effective as energy sources, they should also have this same structure— high carbs, with some good protein and some fat (more fats and oils in winter). A favorite treat of mine in winter is to add a glop of butter to hot chocolate to gain some oomph and add wonderful flavor. If you have food allergies or dietary restrictions, this part of backpacking can be a little more challenging. If you're not allergic to peanuts, one of my favorite trail mixes is composed of dark chocolate peanut M&M's mixed with some other favorite nuts, seeds, and dried fruit, and if you want texture, add some thick-cut rolled oats and puffed millet. With butter mixed in, it also makes a wonderful breakfast. Just add hot water, and *mmmmm*!

Here's an example menu for one of my trips: the above mentioned homemade breakfasts of nuts and oats accompanied by tea or hot chocolate; jerky, potato sticks (like potato chips, except they survive better in a pack), and dark chocolate for lunches; a nut mix with ginger and often more chocolate for snacks; and high-carb and high-protein freeze-dried or home-dried dinners with miso soup and herbal tea for dinners. I have not listed any breads, tortillas, cheese, or noodles; I'm gluten- and generally dairy-intolerant, so I must create a menu that works without those wonderful foods. (Sometimes I cheat and include butter, but I can't do more than that.) This means I can save some weight from not taking these foods, but often have to take other weight to get proper nutrition.

## TO DRINK IS TO LIVE

Water and hydration are part of nutrition. With only a few exceptions, all water in the backcountry these days must be filtered or purified. When I was a kid, we would drink from any mountain stream without fear. Unfortunately, today every wild stream is probably infected with giardia, cryptosporidium, and other not-so- friendly species. Filter or purify all wild water just to be safe. For many years I've used a ceramic MiniWorks pump filter. This works everywhere, is field cleanable, always super reliable, and needs minimal maintenance. But it weighs 16 ounces. So I tried out the Sawyer Squeeze Filter, touted at 3 ounces. (Later I found out that the filter weighs 3 ounces, but if you include the 2-liter water bottle required to use it, the syringe for backflushing, and a tiny towel needed to be sure tainted water does not pollute the clean water, it weighs some 7 ounces. This year the company has come out with a newer version of the filter that weighs 2 ounces, but the same accoutrements are required.) This saves 10 ounces over the ceramic filter, and packs very small. It can be expected to work in lots of conditions, although I have only used it in fairly benign streams. This is a great improvement.

But to really enter the ultralight world here, we need to embrace Aquamira liq- uid water-purification drops. These are a miracle in two tiny bottles (the two 1-ounce

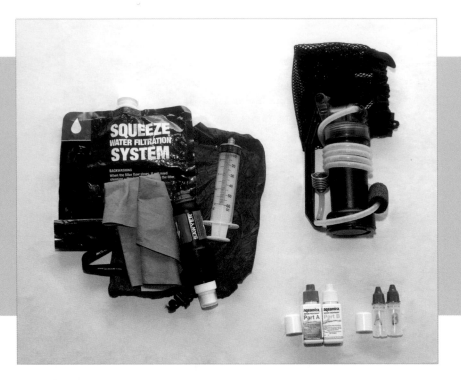

bottles clean some 30 gallons of water). I repackage these into my own tinier bottles, so I carry less than 1 ounce for 30 liters of purified water. They increase the oxygen in the water so it not only kills everything bad, but it actually makes the water taste better! Super easy to use. You just fill a water bottle from the stream and add seven drops of each of the two components per liter. Wait 30 minutes and it's ready. (By the way, don't forget to turn the container upside down and "bleed" the lid to allow the Aquamira to clean the threads and lid.) If water is murky or filled with particulates, scoop it up in a bucket and add a bit of alum to settle the dirt out before you fill your bottle. Alternatively, you can prefilter the water using a coffee filter or bandana.

(A nutritional note here: Drinking chemicals through water purification over long periods of time can be unhealthy. So if your trek entails backpacking for months on end, I recommend using a filter of some sort rather than chemicals for the duration. Certainly, I would have Aquamira or chlorine dioxide tablets along as a backup, but for trips longer than a week or two, I would definitely use a pump or squeeze system even though it will be heavier to carry.)

In my conventional backpack, I always packed the MiniWorks filter as a separate item. In my ultralight setup, the Aquamira bottles are so small that at first I worried I might lose them in my pack! The fix was simple. Because they are no longer an item to be packed individually, I pack them in my repair kit, and I always know where they are.

For drinking methods, a hydration system such as a bladder and tube will provide more hydration to your body than using water bottles, mostly because we can sip every few minutes from a bladder, and generally we only stop to drink from a bottle every hour or so when we need a rest. Some folks love bladders and some hate them. And, to date, scientific studies on hydration have not supported either approach. For me, the bladder approach seems to work best, and I've found that as long as I only use water in the bladder (no juices or electrolyte mixes, and so on), and I dry the entire thing between hikes, I never have mold problems with the bladder, the tube, or my hydration. Then, when necessary, I bring along a small water bottle for hot chocolate, electrolyte mixes, tea, or any other drinks I want on the trip. By the way, today's collapsible water bottles work as well as traditional Nalgene water bottles but are much lighter weight. If you want a wide-mouth

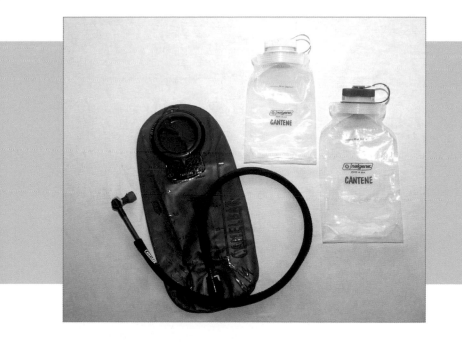

version, Nalgene "collapsible canteens" are the answer. In addition, although the ultralight approach is to use cheap water bottles such as bottled water containers, I find my Camelbak to be more durable and reliable and worth the extra ounces for the ease of hydration it provides. This is a bridge decision that, for me, is worth it because my trips are not about covering as many miles as physically possible, but rather are for enjoyment and fun. Minimizing frustration and making things easy to use are part of my approach. Bladders fit into this category for me. (Of course there are other brands of bladder hydration systems in addition to Camelbak. Choose the one that meets your needs the best.)

## Quick Tips

 Choose the lightest foods that will supply you with the nutrition you need. That includes trail snacks, three meals per day, and possibly snacks in camp, along with some contingency food. For me that's about 1.5 pounds of food per day.

 Remember that backpacking requires more calories than daily life does, in general. This is not the time to skimp on food in order to lose weight.

✓ Collapsible canteens work well as water containers for camp. They pack small and light yet provide ample carrying and storage capacity for water in camp and overnight.

✓ Hydration systems (bladders with hoses) seem to keep us better hydrated on the trail than water bottles, since we tend to sip from the tube often and only stop once in a while for a drink from a bottle. For this reason they are worth the extra weight.

*These are bagpipes. I understand the inventor of the bagpipes was inspired when he saw a man carrying an indignant, asthmatic pig under his arm. Unfortunately, the man-made sound never equalled the purity of the sound achieved by the pig.*

—ALFRED HITCHCOCK

# The Specialty-Gear System

THIS SYSTEM IS INCLUDED for those trips requiring special equipment. Backcountry ski trips, canyoneering treks, rock climbing in the middle of a trek: all of these require us to take specific gear that is normally not included in a regular backpacking trip. Having this system in our list ensures that we don't forget what we need, and that we choose the right pack, shelter, sleeping system, and other gear that meets the requirements of the trip.

Ultralight impacts for this system can be considerable, especially because climbing gear and snowshoes or other winter gear can weigh a lot (see "Winter Considerations," page 95). The choice of pack, as well as the clothing taken on these trips, must be adjusted to handle the extra weight, rigors, and expected conditions. Some specialty gear can be very heavy. For example, the entire philosophy of ultralight comes into question if 20–30 pounds of climbing gear must be carried, making the overall pack weight grow from 20 pounds to perhaps more than 50 pounds! Under such conditions, a conventional pack with a heavier support system may be a better choice than an ultralight pack. And, it may need to be a larger volume pack than your ultralight pack as well.

Some questions to consider:

⚙ Can an ultralight pack accommodate the equipment required for the trip (both in volume and comfort)?

⚙ Are extra clothing layers required for cold weather?

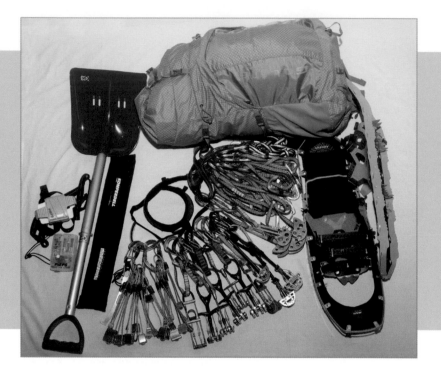

⚙  Will an ultralight shelter, sleeping bag, and pad system accommodate the conditions expected?

⚙  Are snowshoes or skis needed?

✿  *Is carrying snowshoes or skis on the pack required?*

⚙  Is an ice axe required? Ice tools or crampons?

✿  *Are ropes, harness, helmet, and so on, also needed?*

⚙  Are dry bags required?

⚙  Are ropes required for crossing rivers or streams?

⚙  Are extra shoes required for crossing rivers or streams?

⚙  Is any extra gear required to help others who are on the trip?

⚙  Is climbing gear needed?

- *Will you be canyoneering?*
  - What is the canyon rating?
  - Is water expected? Are water shoes required?
  - Are you rappelling only? Ascending also?
  - Will you be doing single-rope rappels?
  - Is contingency gear required?
  - Are any guided rappels required?
  - How many ropes are needed?
    - *Canyoneering or climbing ropes? What length(s)?*
  - Are anchors expected? Extra slings, rap rings, or quick links needed?
  - Will you be canyoneering with full pack or day pack?
  - Will you need a full harness or swami belt?
- *What climbing is expected?*
  - Multi-pitch?
  - Rappelling only?
  - Rock, ice, mixed, glacier?
  - Sport climbing?
  - Trad climbing? Full rack required?
  - What harness will suffice?
  - Is a helmet required?
  - What length of rope is required?
  - Are you climbing with full pack or day pack?
  - Will you be lowering packs over cliffs? Will you be zip-lining packs over pools of water or other obstacles? How long of a line is necessary? Are pulleys needed?

## Quick Tip

✓ Ultralight packs and even bridge packs may not work well if heavy gear is required for a specific activity (like rock climbing or backcountry skiing, where carrying heavy gear in or on the pack is necessary). A conventional pack may be better suited for such cases.

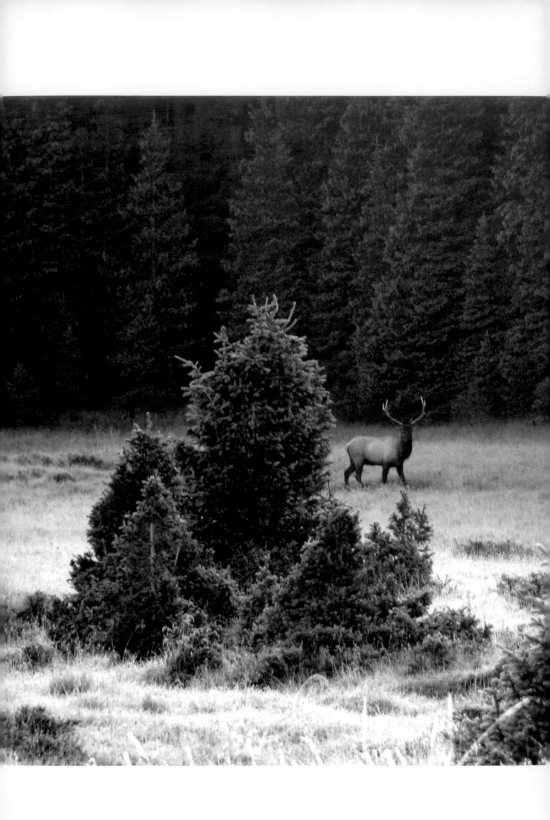

*I wonder if the snow loves the trees and fields, that it kisses them so gently? And then it covers them up snug, you know, with a white quilt; and perhaps it says, "Go to sleep, darlings, till the summer comes again."*

—LEWIS CARROLL

## CHAPTER **5**

# **Winter Considerations**

WINTER TRIPS ARE REALLY FUN AND VERY REWARDING if one is well prepared and knowledgeable in how to function safely and happily in these conditions. Winter backpacking usually requires extra gear, including warmer layers and sleeping bag, more insulation under your sleeping bag, and a much more robust kind of shelter. All of this adds up to more weight. Does the bridging approach to backpacking still apply in the winter? If so, how can we apply these techniques to winter trips?

First, we must define what we mean by winter. In my world, winter includes lots of snow: cold, crisp, fluffy, sparkling, gorgeous blankets of deep white powder. The snow can be fluffy or very wet and heavy. Winter means hiking and camping in the snow with average outside temperatures ranging from some –20°F to a high of maybe 20°F. For most backpackers, storms in winter can create more dangerous conditions than the average summer storms, so these must also be taken into account.

The margin for error is smaller in winter conditions for all wilderness activities, and backpacking is no exception. When we explore the key planning elements for winter trips, we must consider:

- ⚙ the important differences from three-season backpacking,

- ⚙ how we need to modify our thinking and gear organization from that which works the rest of the year, and

- ⚙ what bridging principles can be used to lighten winter loads while preserving safety.

Let's consider these by looking at the gear most impacted by winter conditions.

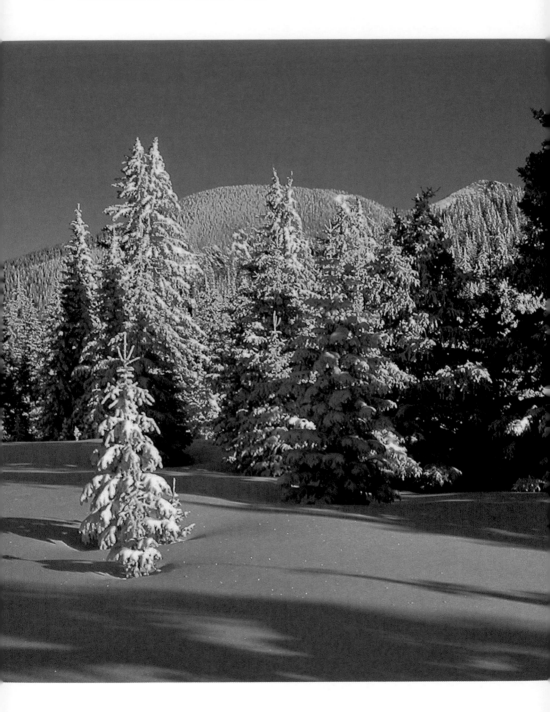

*There's no such thing as bad weather, only unsuitable clothing.*

—ALFRED WAINWRIGHT

# Winter Clothing and Layers

ONE OF MY FIRST WINTER CAMPING TRIPS was to the top of Wolf Creek Pass in southern Colorado, where the snow depth was more than 7 feet under foot. We built an igloo to sleep in, along with snow benches and platforms for cooking. It was pretty fancy. I was cold and wet, but the leaders of this trip were so experienced and inspired by winter camping that they had made their own clothes and sleeping bags out of 1-inch open-cell foam covered in rip stop nylon. They had pants, shirts, booties, mittens, hats. Everything was out of this nylon-covered foam, and they were naked underneath. This approach kept them warm and dry, and thereby kept them happy and healthy in very cold conditions. However, most of us do not use this approach, so we need to think differently about the layers of clothing we use.

The clothes we wear in winter are obviously different from summer wear. Yet there are some overlaps. When I go to the Grand Canyon or to Colorado high country, I always have my down jacket and insulated pants with me. The weather there can change so dramatically in March or November that I must be prepared for almost-winter adventures.

The principles behind layering include the maintenance of core temperature, maximizing comfort, and the wise management of skin temperatures. In the cold of winter (just as in very hot summers), the application of these becomes the central driver behind what clothes we take. In winter, keeping dry and warm can make the difference not only between fun and suffering, but also, potentially, in our survival. The layers we take for three-season backpacking trips also apply here but are modified slightly to handle the winter conditions. Weight is still important, but for many of us, warmth overrides weight, leading to a heavier pack in the end. Here are the three-season layers we discussed earlier, with winter modifications:

- ⚙ **Wicking base layer:** non-cotton T-shirt or, for winter, a long-sleeve base layer

- ⚙ **Wicking and warmer mid-layer:** often windproof but not waterproof fleece, down, or synthetic or possibly a nylon shell with microfleece inside (often no change here for winter)

- ⚙ **Very warm outer layer:** puffy down or the like; again not waterproof, but much warmer and sized to fit over all of the above (Lighter or even ultralight down jackets work for three-season use, but a heavier winter-weight down parka may be called for to handle winter conditions. Today's synthetic expedition jackets might be appropriate here, too, but often are heavier. But those that are both warm and waterproof replace both the down puffy and the waterproof rain-jacket layers, so their weight might even be better than separate layers.)

- ⚙ **Waterproof rain jacket:** waterproof, breathable, lightweight uninsulated outer shell that fits over all of the above (For winter, I use a heavier weight shell that is warmer and more windproof than the ultralight version I use the rest of the year. It is also more abrasion resistant.)

In winter I take heavier gloves and mittens that are waterproof, along with the ski hat and neck gaiter that I take on all trips. The importance of moisture management is amplified in winter, which affects leg and feet warmth considerably. Extra pairs of dry socks are paramount, and the pants I use are heavier for winter.

In summer we are wearing shorts or zip-off pants. In winter, layering dictates different choices for pants to meet my needs. I run a bit hot when carrying a pack, so I don't wear long underwear under hiking pants while trekking in the winter. Rather, I wear my normal three-season hiking pants with a full-featured insulating layer over them. This allows me to take the insulation off during transportation to and from the trailhead, to put it on when necessary or remove it when not, and to vent while hiking via side zips. In addition, I can choose how heavy of a layer to wear.

- ⚙ Lightweight, soft-shell, water-resistant, and breathable pants over my hiking pants (or base layer) are often enough when I am schlepping a full pack uphill.

- ⚙ Warmer, full-side-zip, insulated down pants can be added when it gets really cold.

⚙   Waterproof, breathable rain pants can go over the above for protection from moisture and wind.

   Some of my friends use a base layer under their soft-shell pants instead of hiking pants. It's a matter of personal preference and how hot your body gets when hiking. The important thing for both torso and limbs is to make sure you are warm enough to have full functionality from your muscles and joints without overheating while you exercise. Getting too hot causes excessive sweat, making your skin wet and prone to chill. Again, wicking fabrics are key to manage this moisture effectively. Take off layers or add layers as needed to manage your body temperatures wisely. Never allow the pressure of the group to keep going to interfere with your wise management of your own health needs.

   In winter I often use ski socks instead of summer hiking socks. Today's ski socks are taller, warmer, and made in high-tech designs that manage moisture well. They work to keep my shins warm, and that's where snow is most likely to come in contact with my legs. These in combination with tall gaiters ensure that my

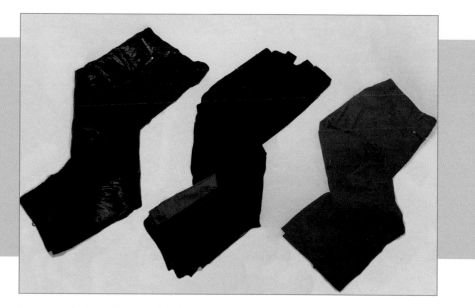

Your metabolism dictates what layers will work best.

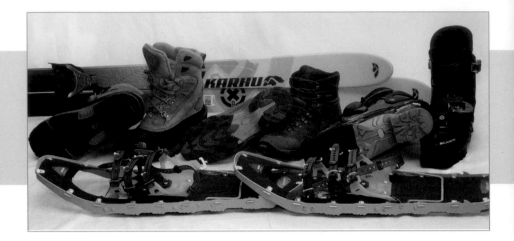

shins, ankles, and feet are properly dressed for snow travel. My summer backpacking boots are also appropriate for much winter travel, as they have a waterproof, breathable membrane in them to keep the wet out. The only issue is ensuring that my feet stay warm. For long hikes, this is usually not a problem when I am moving. It's only in camp that the problem arises. (I could opt for insulated boots with removable liners, but these are often heavier than my Zamberlans and often not all that much warmer.) The cold-feet issue is handled by changing socks upon settling down in camp. Sometimes using a powder spray antiperspirant on my feet also can help to keep my feet drier inside my socks. In addition, if necessary, once in camp sometimes I place a set of oven-baking plastic bags (like Reynolds Oven Bags—not the turkey size but the smaller ones) over my dry feet inside my dry socks inside my boots. This can help keep my feet a good deal warmer.

For short overnight trips, I use a chemical Mega Warmer (made by Grabber) in my boots overnight so I wake up to warm dry boots instead of ice-cold boots to put on my feet in the morning. And I prefer this to putting wet, cold boots inside my sleeping bag. The Mega Warmers are heavy by ultralight standards, weighing 4 ounces each, so I only use them when they will be truly beneficial. However, these air-activated heat pads last 12 hours and work really well for this purpose or as contingency equipment. They also can be used in a sleeping bag or jacket or elsewhere as needed. Sometimes I'll bring an insulated food bag, the kind sold for carrying frozen food home from the store. Using this bag to insulate boots and water bottles, along with a chemical warmer overnight, works extremely well.

For shorter trips or building igloos, when I'm traveling on snowshoes, I have used insulated winter boots (such as Sorrels or North Face Baltoro boots) instead of my hiking boots. These are very comfortable for standing around in the snow for hours, but for me they are not as supportive for long-distance snowshoe hikes with full packs, especially in rough terrain, so I use my hiking boots for longer trips. For ski-based trips, I use boots that fit my backcountry ski bindings. They are insulated and work well, and can even be comfortable for hanging out in camp as long as I loosen them once we arrive at camp. Because skis are not as nimble as snowshoes once in camp, especially when building snow shelters, most of my winter backpacks involve snowshoes.

Bottom line for bridge-packing clothes for winter is that warmth overrides weight, and moisture management must be taken seriously to ensure proper body temperature.

 ## Quick Tips

✓ Layering for winter is really an extension of what you already do for the other seasons. For winter, moisture management is paramount to avoid serious consequences.

✓ Moisture management is not just sweat management, but also ensuring you stay dry while living in the snow.

✓ Contingency planning must include how to stay warm when your original plans fail.

*When the girl returned, some hours later, she carried a tray, with a cup of fragrant tea steaming on it; and a plate piled up with very hot buttered toast, cut thick, very brown on both sides, with the butter running through the holes in great golden drops, like honey from the honeycomb. The smell of that buttered toast simply talked to Toad, and with no uncertain voice; talked of warm kitchens, of breakfasts on bright frosty mornings, of cozy parlour firesides on winter evenings, when one's ramble was over and slippered feet were propped on the fender, of the purring of contented cats, and the twitter of sleepy canaries.*

—KENNETH GRAHAME

## Hydration, Food, and Stoves

HYDRATION AND FOOD provide us with the energy to create heat, which is, of course, what we need to enjoy winter, and more than that, to stay alive in harsh winter conditions. Often in winter, when it's cold, we don't drink as much as we do when it's a hot summer day. Alas, that is the opposite of what we need to stay warm! And, drinking enough can be tricky in winter since water tends to freeze. As important as food and water are in the summer, they must be planned even more carefully for winter treks.

Drinking from a hydration system (like a Camelbak bladder and tube or equivalent) hydrates us better than water bottles alone. This is still true in the winter. The problem many people encounter is frozen tubes or bite valves. Here's what I recommend to prevent the water from freezing:

- If dealing with extreme cold, fill the bladder with warm or hot water. This is expensive in fuel usage, but may be necessary.

- Blow into the bite valve to push water back into the bladder after every drink. This prevents water from freezing in the tube.

- ⚙ Store the bite valve inside the front of your shirt next to your skin, stuffing the tube down inside the neck of your shirt a bit. This simple trick prevents the valve from freezing.

- ⚙ At night, be sure to close the lock on your bite valve then put the entire bladder and hose into your sleeping bag to keep it warm. You can put the entire thing into a large baggie and seal it if you want insurance in case of a leak.

If you choose to take water bottles instead of a hydration system, be sure to pack the bottles upside down and preferably in insulating bottle holders or clothes inside the pack. Turning the bottle upside down prevents the water from freezing to the cap.

Water purification in winter is simple: Just melt snow. When melting the snow, you do not need to boil it, but you can if you feel it has been compromised. Be sure to put some water into the pot along with the snow before you turn on the stove. This prevents the pot from burning and saves fuel. If you are camping where there is not enough snow to melt for drinking water, then life becomes more complex. Stream water needs purification. Chlorine dioxide tablets work well, are light in weight, don't freeze, and save the fuel required to bring water to a boil. Aquamira drops work wonderfully in non-winter months but can freeze, so they are not the best choice for winter trips. They still can be used, however, as long as you are careful to ensure the bottles stay warm (perhaps in your pocket next to your body). The ultralight trade-offs here are (1) the weight of fuel for boiling versus tablets (one tablet per liter) or drops, and (2) the means to carry water while hiking, which might be different from what you use in the summer.

As for food, cooking, and stoves, the same ultralight principles apply; however, in winter we need more calories to keep us warm. So plan meals that include some butter, oil, nuts, or other foods that are high in fat. In addition, plan meals that are easy to prepare with just boiled water, such as freeze-dried dinners. These minimize weight. Since fuel is limited, we don't want to waste it for heating dishwater. Meals that can be eaten out of the bag or in a cup that can then be used for tea or soup allow us to dirty only one dish that is almost self-cleaning (via the tea or soup), or at least easier to clean up with snow after dinner.

Since our meals require only boiling water, the stove and pot we bring should be oriented toward melting snow. A larger pot on a very efficient wind-resistant stove is recommended. Canister systems like the MSR Reactor stove with integrated pot (especially the new 2.5-liter version), or possibly the Jetboil Sumo, offer superior performance to generic stoves that are susceptible to wind and not as efficient in heat transfer. The Reactor is the best choice among these because it is fully windproof. I also have used the MSR Windpro II stove with a larger aluminum or titanium pot. Because it can be protected from the wind and can support the canister upside down, it works well in the cold. In all cases, when using canister stoves be sure to sleep with the canister in your sleeping bag so it will be more efficient in the morning. Liquid-fuel stoves today are less appropriate in winter due to the frustrations inherent in the possible frostbite danger of liquid gas on skin and the improved technology in canister stoves. For many decades this was not the case, and we simply got used to using liquid-gas systems. But today's new stoves have opened up many more choices.

I also recommend bringing a small platform for the stove. This can be a simple piece of lightweight plastic layered onto a scrap of closed-cell foam (or a piece of wood or whatever is lightweight to carry), designed to hold your stove in place so it won't slip off when the platform is wet and uneven, and large enough to hold both the stove and the fuel and possibly your pot when it is not on the stove.

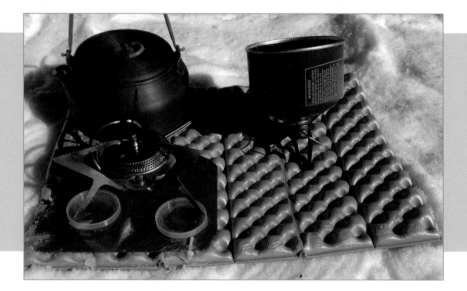

# Quick Tips

✓ Meals in winter must be planned with snow in mind. Hence, target high-calorie, high-carb, and high-protein foods with a higher fat content that are the lightest possible weight.

✓ Hydration methods must survive extreme cold and be easy to use.

✓ Building a lightweight stove platform can make meals more successful and less of a hassle, thereby minimizing frustration and ensuring life-saving nutrition when storm conditions intend otherwise.

Put some bolts through the platform (or other devices), or use a bumpy pad as the base of the platform so it can hold itself in place on the snow. (Picture in your mind using it on a snow shelf upon which you are cooking.) Such a platform can make cooking a delight rather than frustrating. Using closed-cell foam insulates from the snow and thus helps make heating more efficient. The pad also provides an insulated table on which to put your freeze-dried dinners as they cook. If you wrap your SAM splint around the food as an insulating cozy, the cooking is even more efficient. A Thermarest Z-Lite sit pad is a great choice for this foam base. It is the right size and weight, it has dimples that help hold it in place on the snow, and the new models have one silver side to reflect the heat of the stove. Zip-tying some stiffening plastic to this foam (with small plastic cups glued to it to hold the stove in place) makes a wonderful and lightweight kitchen counter!

> *The biggest misconception that people have about winter camping is that it's going to be this cold, awful experience.*
>
> —MATT LLOYD

## Winter Sheltering and Sleeping Systems

SLEEPING UNDER THE STARS is a sublime experience. But in winter, most of us need more shelter than that. (I know a few brave souls who do sleep under the stars in winter, but they are rare indeed!) Can't we just use our three-season tents? Well, it depends. Ultralight shelters often do not provide sufficient shelter for most winter conditions due to the way they handle wind and moisture. Some conventional free-standing tents will work in winter, and their specific design will dictate how well

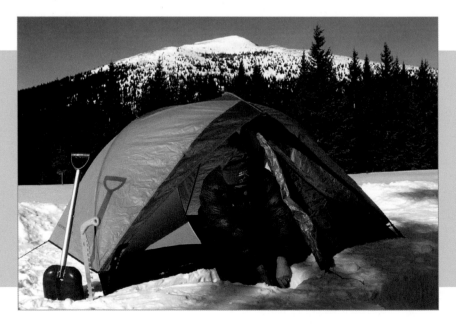

Donning boots at the door of a four-season tent. Note the snow saw and shovel used to create a place to sit.

they will work. Minimizing moisture in the tent is paramount in winter camping. Tents with a lot of mesh close to the ground invite snow into the tent (especially in wind), which then turns into water inside the tent. Tents with closed fabric up the sides of the tent with mesh at the top are better suited for winter use, but not as good as true four-season tents. Freestanding tents are better for winter use, because it is not always guaranteed that you can stake down your shelter sufficiently for a taut pitch. Certainly a snow stake buried as a "dead man" will work well to secure the lines and corners of your tent in most snow conditions, but the setting up and taking down of non-freestanding tents can be messy in snow. Regardless, it is better to use a tent designed for winter, or better still, to build a snow shelter!

Snow shelters are far warmer than tents, provide complete weather coverage, and insulate against sound and light far better than any tent. Snow camping can become the Ritz when your shelter is an igloo or other properly constructed snow shelter. For example, when it's 20°F below zero outside, it will be only slightly warmer than that inside your tent, where in a snow shelter it will be 25°–30°F or

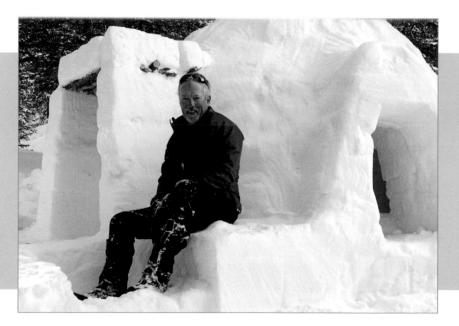

My friend Ash enjoying the porch of a newly completed igloo. Note the gear-storage shed behind him and the door to the interior on the right.

so, consistently, even when it's −20°F outside. Being inside a snow shelter is a "sensory deprivation" experience! It is so completely dark that you cannot tell day from night, and it is almost completely soundproof. A great night's sleep indeed! Bring a tea-candle to set on a small shelf inside the shelter. They weigh very little and will light up the entire shelter and bring you joy and wonderful ambience! (It's also nice to bring a pee bottle for use in the middle of the night. Ahem . . .)

How do snow shelters keep us warmer? Well, snow traps air, and air insulates, just like a down sleeping bag. Eight- to twelve-inch-thick walls trap a lot of air, hence they provide a lot of insulation. They freeze into position and provide solid, stable, and weatherproof protection from high winds, snow storms, cold weather, and, of course, grumpiness. Sleeping in one of these castles is truly delightful if you have the right gear.

A few years ago, my friend Ash and I went up to about 11,000 feet on a nearby ridge for a quick winter overnight. He had a new winter tent he wanted to test, and I wanted to build an igloo. Turned out the snow was not the right consistency to support a full igloo, so we built a snow trench—a shelter composed of a ditch about 3 feet wide and roughly the same in depth, with blocks of snow supporting each other to comprise a roof over the trench. The doorway is at one end of the trench, with an air hole in the roof opposite the door. We had a fun dinner under the stars and went to bed with temperatures expected to drop below zero overnight. He was in his tent, I in my trench. Inside my shelter, I had a tarp on which was my sleeping bag. I installed a tea candle into a notch in the wall to give me wonderful lighting, and proceeded to settle in for the night. Once in bed, I blew out the light and slept. Upon waking I found it was completely dark, silent, and still. I thought it must be midnight or something, but I needed to pee, so I made the effort to get outside. What a surprise! It was 7 a.m., the sun was shining with blue sky above, and Ash was fixing breakfast! The snow trench was so well insulated that it was completely dark and silent even in the bustle of morning. What a great night's sleep!

There are many kinds of snow shelters, ranging from simple depressions in the snow to snow trenches with block-constructed roofs to complete igloos of many types. The latter two of these provide the most warmth and comfort. Snow depressions work in a pinch, but are not for everyone (sleeping under the stars, et al). If you are planning to sleep in a snow shelter that has not yet been built, you must schedule your day such that you have the appropriate time to build the shelter upon your arrival, and you must bring along the necessary tools. An avalanche shovel and probe, along with a snow saw and a tape measure, will give you the tool basis for most block-based construction. Knowing what to do with these tools and how to quickly and efficiently build your shelter is, of course, a necessary prerequisite.

On one hand, sheltering in this way lightens your load, because you only need to bring a tarp to put underneath your sleeping bag. On the other hand, it requires you bring along the tools to build your shelter—unless it's already built ahead of time. (We often do day trips to build igloos and other kinds of snow shelters early in the winter, and then when it's time to use them, we don't need to carry the tools or spend the energy building our home upon our arrival.)

What about the sleeping system? Does it need to change for winter use? It depends! If you are using a tent for your shelter, you will need a winter-rated sleeping system. That means a sleeping bag and pad that can handle serious winter temperatures, often below zero. But if you are in a snow shelter, because the temperature is always around 25°–30°F, you can bring a three-season bag and be fine with a pad that insulates well. (As usual, warmth depends on the food you eat, exercise of the day, your layering, and whether you are a "cold sleeper" or "hot sleeper" as described in the discussion on three-season sleeping systems on page 62.)

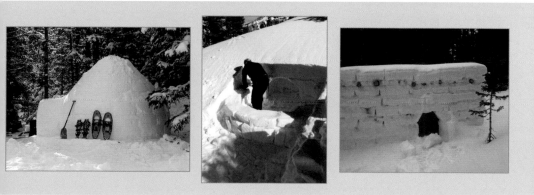

Snow Shelters

The pad for winter cannot be the tiny one that I chose for my ultralight three-season sleeping system. In winter we need full-body insulation under our entire sleeping system. This can be accomplished with a full-length insulating pad or a combination of two shorter pads—for example, a "short" self-inflating 1.5-inch-thick pad for the torso used in conjunction with a "short" ¾-inch-thick closed-cell foam pad for the legs and feet. ("Short" pads are generally 47 inches in length.) This combination allows us to have a pad for use in camp and on the trail (the closed-cell pad), along with warmer and more comfortable padding for the torso when sleeping. The weight of this combination is actually less than many of the full-length pads that have high R-value ratings. Whatever you choose, be sure it insulates well (high R-value) and can handle moisture.

Your sleeping system should also include a warm hat, possibly a neck gaiter, warm dry socks, and full-body base layers. The sleeping bag should have room at the feet to include your clothes from the day (change into sleeping clothes) so the day clothes can dry over night. This is part of the moisture-management regimen that ensures maximum warmth and comfort both day and night. (Yes, we do generate moisture inside our bags at night, but our body heat is enough to dry damp clothes in most cases. The exception, of course, is in high-humidity wet conditions that last for multiple days. You might have to bring extra clothes to handle these conditions.)

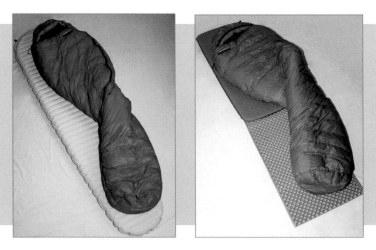

Comparison of Sleeping Pads for Winter

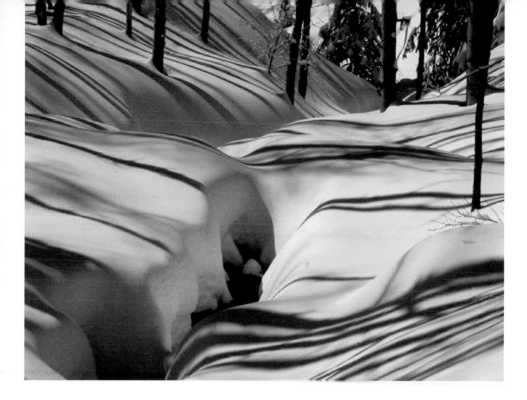

![Quick Tips icon] **Quick Tips**

✓ Winter shelters must be able to handle serious cold and weather conditions. Snow shelters offer the most comfort for the least weight.

✓ Be sure your sleeping system is tailored to the shelter you choose in order to ensure appropriate warmth.

Bottom line: Your sleeping and shelter system in winter might end up weighing about the same as your summer one, or possibly a bit heavier. Super-ultralight shelters and sleeping systems will definitely be lighter but not warm enough for winter use. Heavy conventional gear also will work, but it will be a burden due to its weight. So a bridge system that is tailored to your specific winter-trip styles, personal needs, and the weather and locations of your trips, is again appropriate. And, of course, winter contingency planning generally also adds additional weight. Under some conditions, the bridge pack is not the right choice for a winter trip. This is considered in more detail in the next section.

*Many people do not realize that the snowshoe can be used for a great
many things besides walking on snow. For instance, it can be used to carry
pancakes from the stove to the breakfast table.*

—JACK HANDEY

## Snowshoes and Skis

SOME PLACES ARE accessible in winter without the need for snow flotation, but
most winter treks require boot-traction devices (like Katoola Microspikes or equivalent), snowshoes, or backcountry (or possibly Nordic) skis. This impacts your selection of footwear, because your boots must fit appropriately into whatever you are
using to travel over the snow. Warmth is also an issue, as different kinds of footwear
insulate better or worse than others. Some trips require multiple styles of travel,
dictating the need to carry skis, snowshoes, or Katoolas for all or part of the trip.

This also impacts which pack you take on such trips, because it must support
the carrying of skis or snowshoes on the outside of the pack in a convenient manner. Packs designed for winter treks include a front-access "dry gear" pocket, along
with external support mechanisms for carrying your skis or snowshoes and an

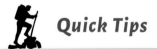 *Quick Tips*

✓ Flotation devices can make a trip much more enjoyable and offer a means to
handle emergency situations (such as creating a stretcher out of skis). Pick the
right kind of flotation for the expected terrain and snow conditions.

✓ Since the pack you pick for winter outings must be able to handle the rigors of
the expected itinerary, ultralight gear may not work if you have to carry skis,
snowshoes, or a snowboard on the pack.

outer "wet gear" pocket for your shovel and probe, et al. Such packs are not in the ultralight category but might be worth choosing due to their increased functionality in winter conditions. Similarly, ultralight packs may not be comfortable enough to support the weight of skis added to the weight of the other gear required, and many ultralight packs do not have the means to support strapping snowshoes or skis onto the pack. Experiment with what you have before embarking on your winter trek to be sure the pack you pick will work appropriately and comfortably.

Furthermore, in addition to how they fit onto the pack, the choice of which kind of ski or snowshoe to take on a specific trek must be related to the chores of the trip. If you are building a snow shelter upon arrival, smaller, more maneuverable snowshoes are more convenient during the shelter construction. Skis, on the other hand, make it faster and easier (usually) to get to and from the end location if the terrain is relatively flat or rolling. Skiing on a known and predefined track can be great with Nordic skis, but often rough, unpacked terrain requires a backcountry ski or equivalent to navigate difficult features. Steep terrain is probably more suited to the use of snowshoes on the way up and skis on the way down (unless you are a novice skier, when snowshoes will be safer going downhill). So again, it depends, but the pack will be lighter if you can take only one flotation method (skis or snowshoes).

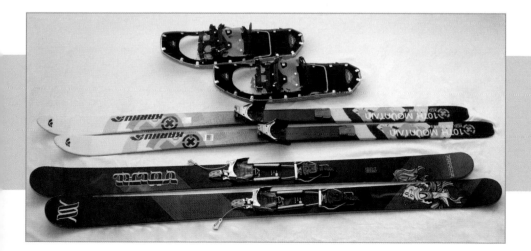

*Adventures are all very well in their place, but there's a lot to be said for regular meals and freedom from pain.*

—NEIL GAIMAN

# Winter Contingency Planning

ALL SERIOUS BACKCOUNTRY trekking requires contingency planning and gear no matter what the season. (For more on this, see "Three-Season Contingency Planning," on page 76). Winter is no exception, but it requires a slightly different set of backup gear items in order to be prepared to handle the unexpected in deep snow and cold. Normally I take more in this category than most ultralight backpackers take, even in summer. That's part of my bridging choice, allowing me to be prepared to handle serious injuries that come unexpectedly. Elsewhere I mention my experience with splinting ankles in the backcountry. I always have my SAM splint along. In the winter, the cold is a huge adversary. Injured people need to be insulated from the snow, insulated from the wind and cold, yet still administered first aid as one might in three-season conditions. This can be a significant challenge, especially in rugged, steep terrain or deep snow. When there is a blizzard on top of this, things really get interesting!

OK, what to take for contingency? I always expect to handle an unexpected overnight, so I have a lightweight emergency bivvy (a lightweight, reinforced reflective Mylar bag, much like an uninsulated sleeping bag, just big enough for a person, that protects from weather and reflects body heat back onto the person inside) and extra warm layers with me. I always have my Z-rest short pad with me to sit on for lunch and to use to insulate an unfortunate victim from the snow. As trip leader, I always carry more hats and gloves and dry socks than I think I will need for myself, and my down jacket or fleece vest can always be used on someone else since I bring extra layers along. Remember that warmth is determined in part by what you eat, so I always have a stove, pot, cup, and soup packets, along with honey-ginger packets to warm someone when needed. I bring ginger since it is known to stimulate circulation, calm nausea, and soothe digestion. It's an excellent contingency food for winter. Hot chocolate is probably worth bringing, even if it's not for contingency! The stove allows the creation of more hydration when needed, as well as the option of hot drinks to warm and provide nutrition.

One last note on contingency planning: These days there is amazing technology available to help us. The use of personal locator beacons can be a godsend in the right conditions (the ACR ResQLink systems, the SPOT Gen III, or the DeLorme InReach SE and Explorer, are the latest available right now). Sometimes these units cannot connect to send a signal, but when they do work, you can notify search and rescue (SAR) of your situation and get help on the way immediately. These units send your exact GPS location so the SAR folks can find you quickly. The InReach units allow two-way texting between you and SAR, so you can let them know the conditions of the injured party for appropriate response. Not all trips require the use of these or warrant the extra weight (or emotional security) they provide. I don't often take one of these, but I have friends who take them on every trip. It's another trade-off.

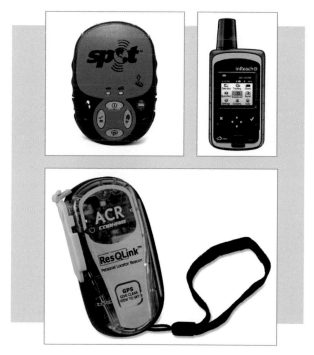

Personal Locator Beacons

## Quick Tips

✓ The margin of error in winter is small. How much extra gear weight are you willing to carry to save a person's life? What about saving your own life if you are injured?

✓ Survival in winter requires not only contingency planning but also knowing a bit about how food creates heat and provides nutrition. Having the perfect extra food along could make all the difference. Plan well.

All of this adds weight. This comes under the category of trip-leader responsibilities and the consideration of how much weight a person's life is worth. Winter is unforgiving, so I try to be prepared for the worst scenario and hope it never happens. (For more on contingency management, see "Assessing and Managing Risk," on page 130.)

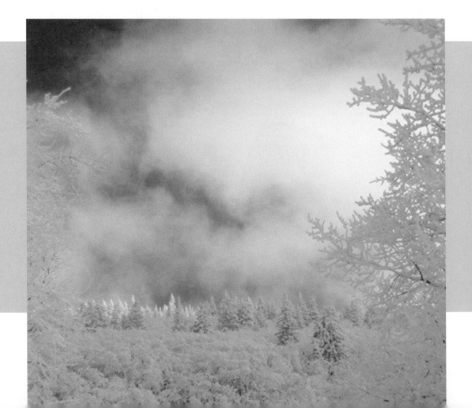

*The real voyage of discovery consists not in seeking new landscapes, but in having new eyes.*

—MARCEL PROUST

# CHAPTER **6**

# Putting It All Together

REMEMBER THE GEAR-ASSESSMENT SPREADSHEET you started at the beginning of this book? Now return to it. Research the replacement items that meet your goals, weight criteria, and comfort. Weigh them and fill in the spreadsheet. If you are savvy with Excel, you can have a box at the bottom that adds up all of your old gear weights and all of the new gear weights, subtracts them, and displays your total weight savings, along with your new total gear weight. If this is everything but food, water, and fuel, this becomes your new base weight.

Notice the "Importance Rating" column. This rating helps reduce the "fluff" in the pack: items that you habitually take because "you might need them" or someone said you "had to have along." If you never use them, don't take them— unless you consciously choose them as part of your contingency plan.

Once you have this chart completed, try reducing the weight of one system by experimenting with new gear. Once you're happy with that system, move to another until you have gone through all nine systems. I did the pack first, then the shelter, then the sleeping system, then the fire and nutrition systems, and so on. (This might not be the best approach. If you do the pack last, you will have a better idea of your total weight, and hence a better idea of what volume and style of pack you need.) By concentrating on one system at a time, it becomes less over-whelming and more cost-effective. Remember, bridging is not only OK, it is the

most effective way to navigate this transition. It's also OK to choose some gear, use it for some years or months, and then repeat this process to reduce weight further.

By the way, in my case, my new pack weight (everything but consumables) has dropped from 27.26 pounds to 14.89 pounds, bringing my base weight (total weight less winter clothes and chair) down to 11.29 pounds. So I get to carry *12.37 fewer pounds* for every trip from now on! And, I'm still a comfortable sleeper, a happy hiker, completely self-sufficient, and able to cook any meals I like. This weight does not take into account additional group gear that might be required on some trips; plus, this is for three-season trips, not winter backpacking trips, which require extra gear (see "Winter Considerations," page 95, for more details).

An 11.29-pound base weight is not the 8.5 pounds that I dreamed about. But for a bridge setup, coming from my conventional base weight, it's fantastic! This result is also realistic, functional, and attainable—not only for me, but for you, too!

Turn the page for some sample weight comparisons between conventional gear and ultralight bridge choices.

 ## Quick Tips

✓ Thinking modularly organizes your gear and simplifies this process. Think of each module as a system of gear that accomplishes one specific task (sleeping, eating, and so on).

✓ Be very clear about what your requirements are, then choose the lightest gear that meets those requirements.

## SAMPLE WEIGHT COMPARISONS

| GEAR TYPE | CONVENTIONAL CHOICE AND WEIGHT | BRIDGE CHOICE AND WEIGHT |
|---|---|---|
| **1. HIKING SYSTEM** | | |
| ✦ Pack | ✦ Gregory Baltoro 70 **91 oz.** | ✦ GoLite Jam 50 **28.7 oz.** |
| ✦ Rain cover for pack | ✦ Sea to Summit Large **4.4 oz.** | ✦ Gregory 50L **2.9 oz.** |
| ✦ Camelbak bladder, collapsible water bottles | ✦ Camelbak + 48-oz. Nalgene canteen **10 oz.** | ✦ (No replacement necessary) **10 oz.** |
| ✦ Chair | | |
| ✦ 30-foot cord, bear bag stuff sack, extra straps, and so on | ✦ REI Flexlite **26.4 oz.** (included in repair kit) | ✦ (No replacement necessary) **26.4 oz.** |
| **2. CLOTHING SYSTEM** | | |
| ✦ Raincoat | ✦ REI Ultralight coat **12.2 oz.** | ✦ Outdoor Research Helium 2 **6.2 oz.** |
| ✦ Rain pants | ✦ Marmot Precip pants **11.3 oz.** | ✦ Zpacks Cuben Fiber pants **3.5 oz.** |
| ✦ Hats, gloves, neck gaiter | ✦ (Misc.) **5.1 oz.** | ✦ (No replacement necessary) **5.1 oz.** |
| ✦ Down jacket | ✦ Mountain Hardwear Phantom **16 oz.** | ✦ Feathered Friends Hyperion **12.4 oz.** |
| ✦ Mid-layer jacket | ✦ Marmot windshirt **15.9 oz.** | ✦ Marmot Stride jacket **9.9 oz.** |
| ✦ Insulated pants | ✦ Patagonia Nanopuff pants **17.4 oz.** | ✦ Montbell UL TEC Down pants **13.7 oz.** |
| **3. SHELTER, SLEEPING, AND LIGHTING SYSTEM** | | |
| ✦ Tent | ✦ MSR Hubba tent, footprint, stakes **62.2 oz.** | ✦ Zpacks Hexamid Solo Plus, footprint, stakes **23.3 oz.** |
| ✦ Sleeping bag | ✦ Marmot Helium (30-degree) **26.7 oz.** | ✦ Feathered Friends Hummingbird (20-degree) **26.6 oz.** |
| ✦ Silk liner | ✦ Cocoon Silk mummy **4.5 oz.** | ✦ (Not needed with new sleeping bag) |
| ✦ Pillow or pillowcase | ✦ Thermarest Synthetic pillow **7.2 oz.** | ✦ Exped UL Airpillow **1.4 oz.** |
| ✦ Sleeping pad | ✦ Thermarest Prolite Plus short **16 oz.** | ✦ Klymit Inertia X-lite **7.3 oz.** |
| ✦ Headlamp and extra batteries, and/or extra headlamp | ✦ Black Diamond Spot + older lamp **5.1 oz.** | ✦ Fenix HL21 + extra battery **3 oz.** |

## SAMPLE WEIGHT COMPARISONS *(continued)*

| GEAR TYPE | CONVENTIONAL CHOICE AND WEIGHT | BRIDGE CHOICE AND WEIGHT |
|---|---|---|
| **3. SHELTER, SLEEPING, AND LIGHTING SYSTEM** *(continued)* | | |
| ✦ Pee bottle | ✦ 32-oz. Nalgene canteen **2 oz.** | ✦ (No replacement necessary) **2 oz.** |
| **4. NAVIGATION SYSTEM** | | |
| ✦ Compass | ✦ Mirrored field compass **2.3 oz.** | ✦ Small generic compass **0.4 oz.** |
| **5. FIRST-AID, REPAIR, AND PERSONAL-HYGIENE SYSTEM** | | |
| ✦ First-aid kit | ✦ Large homemade kit + SAM splint **33 oz.** | ✦ Smaller homemade kit + SAM splint **24.2 oz.** |
| ✦ Repair kit | ✦ Large homemade one with bivvy **22 oz.** | ✦ Smaller homemade one, still with bivvy **15.4 oz.** |
| ✦ Toiletries and zip-top bags for packing out used TP | ✦ Homemade **5.5 oz.** | ✦ (No replacement necessary) **5.5 oz.** |
| ✦ Tiny towel | ✦ Older Cascade Designs model **1.4 oz.** | ✦ Modern small REI towel **1 oz.** |
| **6. COMMUNICATION SYSTEM** | | |
| ✦ Signal mirror, whistle | ✦ (Not included because often not taken) | ✦ (Not included because often not taken) |
| ✦ Two-way radios | ✦ (Not included because often not taken) | ✦ (Not included because often not taken) |
| **7. FIRE AND NUTRITION SYSTEMS** | | |
| ✦ Knife | ✦ Buck Redpoint knife **2.8 oz.** | ✦ Razor blade **0.1 oz.** |
| ✦ Stove | ✦ MSR Windpro II **11.6 oz.** | ✦ Soto Windmaster **2.7 oz.** |
| ✦ Cooking pot(s) | ✦ MSR Haulite Aluminum Tea Pot **6 oz.** | ✦ REI Ti large cup **3.3 oz.** |
| ✦ Water filter | ✦ MSR Miniworks ceramic filter **15.9 oz.** | ✦ Aquamira drops **1 oz.** |
| ✦ Spoon and cup | ✦ Aluminum spoon, Ti cup **2.3 oz.** | ✦ (No replacement necessary) **2.3 oz.** |
| **TOTAL WEIGHT** | **Conventional Gear:** 436.2 oz. = 27.26 lb. | **Bridge Gear:** 238.3 oz. = 14.89 lb. |

*Method is like packing things in a box; a good packer will get in half as much again as a bad one.*

—EDWARD CHRISTIAN DAVID GASCOYNE, LORD CECIL

# Packing to Minimize Frustration

**AT FIRST GLANCE,** it seems that filling the pack with gear should be effortless: Just dump in the stuff and go. But anyone who has carried such a pack knows that is a big mistake. A well-organized and well-balanced pack can be a joy to carry. On the other hand, carrying a poorly packed one can be very uncomfortable and frustrating. Although there are differences in how to pack between conventional and ultralight packs, the central principles are the same. (Later in this chapter I show examples of how to pack both conventional and bridge packs. Refer to "Gear Organization," page 28, for ideas on how to create easy-to-pack systems.)

These are the main principles involved in achieving a joy-to-use pack:

⚙ **Everything goes inside the pack.**

  ✦  Choose an internal-frame pack.

  ✦  Only extremely bulky items like a closed-cell foam pad go on the outside of the pack.

⚙ **Balance the pack.**

  ✦  Organize weight inside the pack so the center of balance is close to your own center of balance.

  ✦  Pack heaviest items close to your spine, between the small of your back and your shoulder blades. This is why hydration bladder sleeves are located where they are, to place that heavy water weight in that sweet spot close to your spine.

  ✦  Lighter items inside the pack go on the bottom, sides, and top, surrounding the heavier items in the middle.

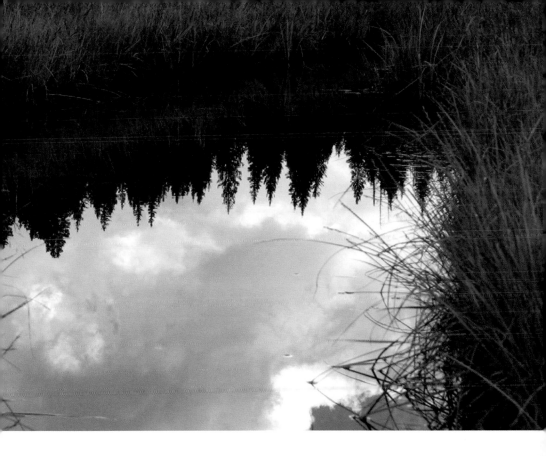

⚙ **Tall items** like tent poles, fishing poles, or chairs can be placed into the front corners of the pack, standing along the vertical axis near the frame of the pack so they are out of the way.

✦ Organize items in the pack so the pack is balanced side-to-side.

✦ The drawing on page 125 shows how to balance the load practically.

⚙ **Keep in mind ease of packing, unpacking, and use of the pack contents.**

✦ Logical organization of gear minimizes frustration in the backcountry.

✦ Pack gear modularly. Organize your gear into systems and pack each system into one stuff sack.

✦ Pack according to when items will be needed: Items not needed until camp can go on the bottom; items needed en route should be at the top or in outside pockets. Lunch and jackets that might be needed en route should be accessible. Pack your shelter near the top of the pack in case it is raining when you need to set up camp.

✦ No space is wasted.

⚙ **Pack for stability.**

✦ Nothing should move during transit. As you walk, the pack is stable and centered, riding well and close to your back. It moves with you and does not cause you to be off balance as you hike. Nothing flops, dangles, wobbles, or shifts.

⚙ **Pack for comfort.**

✦ The pack should be sized and fit properly to the torso of the hiker. Poor fit will greatly impact not only function of the pack suspension but also the overall comfort of the pack during use.

✦ The pack must be properly adjusted to transfer the weight appropriately to the bones of the legs.

✦ The table on page 126 shows how to size, fit, and adjust a pack.

*A note about stuff sacks:* Some of my friends never use stuff sacks when backpacking, choosing instead to cram items into the pack at random so as to most efficiently use the nooks and crannies between items inside the pack. I prefer to use modular packing systems and a small number of stuff sacks. By appropriately mixing the soft and squishy items with harder items, I end up not having many nooks left to fill. Certainly, one can use too many stuff sacks and end up adding unnecessary weight. However, if carefully thought out, one can end up with around half a dozen stuff sacks plus a couple of food bags (main storage and lunch), and thereby increase orderliness in the pack, minimize the possibilities of losing gear, and maximize the ease of packing, unpacking, and finding gear when you need it. For most of these, I prefer ultralight Ultrasil nylon sacks with zippers along the side. Obviously, this and the modular systems you choose fall into the category of personal preferences.

In a frameless or ultralight pack, it is important not to pack hard items like cooking pots or fuel canisters next to the hiker's spine. Place softer, more pliable items along the hiker's back.

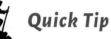 **Quick Tip**

✓ Pack to minimize frustration. This allows us to quickly find things when we need them while minimizing weight, maximizing balance in the pack, and facilitating the use of our gear. All of this increases the probability of having more fun on trips.

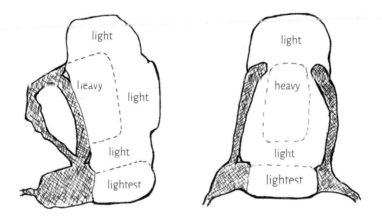

How to Balance Gear Inside the Pack

To determine if a pack fits you well, perform the following steps with a weighted, properly packed pack that is approximately the right torso length for you.

## HOW TO SIZE, FIT, AND ADJUST A PACK

| | |
|---|---|
| 1. | Loosen all adjustment straps, making sure all compression straps are snug and tight. |
| 2. | Load the pack onto your back. |
| 3. | Secure the hip belt snugly, making sure that it is centered vertically on the top of the iliac crest (the belt should straddle the top of the hip bone, aligned under the armpit). Then tighten load-stabilizer straps firmly (if your pack has these). |
| 4. | Tighten shoulder-harness straps until buckles are aligned with seams under armpits; then tighten a tiny bit more (just slightly overtighten for now). |
| 5. | Gently pull down and forward on the load-lifter straps just until the weight moves to the hips and no more. |
| 6. | Loosen the shoulder-harness straps slightly to align them again to the underarm seam (roughly centered at seam under armpit, about halfway between pit and hip belt). You should feel about 80–85% of the weight on the hips and 15–20% on the shoulders at this time, and the pack should feel comfortable. You might need to loosen shoulder-harness straps to achieve this distribution of weight. |
| 7. | Fasten sternum strap and adjust for comfort; this should just be snug, not too tight. |
| 8. | Shoulder harnesses should form a smooth curve over the shoulders, with possibly a small gap (just large enough for your pinky) behind the top of the shoulder. (Look in a mirror to see the curve over the shoulders.) Large gaps or "pooches" are indications that the harness is the wrong size or needs adjustment. The shoulder straps should meet the pack body approximately 1.5–2 inches vertically below the top of the shoulder. If this distance is too large, the pack needs to be adjusted if possible, and if it cannot be adjusted, the pack is too small for your torso length. And if this distance is very small or the straps meet the pack body above the shoulder, the pack torso length is too long for your back, and the load-lifters will not do their job. |
| 9. | The goal is to feel the weight in the legs. The pack itself should be almost transparently present. There should be no uncomfortable pressure points. If these exist, the fit is wrong or needs major adjustment, or this is the wrong pack for your body. |

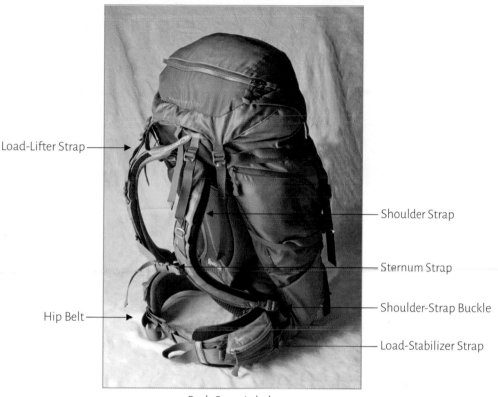

Load-Lifter Strap

Shoulder Strap

Sternum Strap

Hip Belt

Shoulder-Strap Buckle

Load-Stabilizer Strap

Pack-Strap Labels
*(see table opposite for uses)*

The next two pages demonstrate how to balance your gear to create a well-organized pack. One set of illustrations is for conventional gear, the other for a bridge pack. Although the principles are the same, there are distinct differences in how the two packs are loaded, mostly due to the structure of each pack and the smaller size and weight of the ultralight gear.

# PACKING LAYERS

| Conventional | Bridge |
|:---:|:---:|

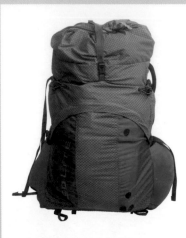

## LAYER 1

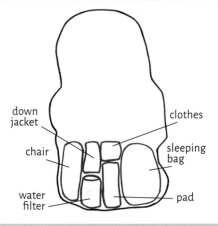

down
jacket

chair

water
filter

clothes

sleeping
bag

pad

down
pants

chair

down
jacket

## LAYER 2

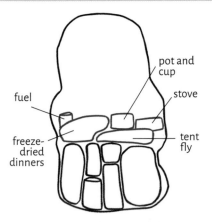

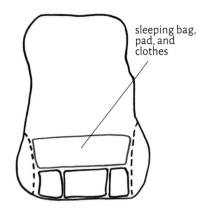

pot and
cup

fuel

stove

freeze-
dried
dinners

tent
fly

sleeping bag,
pad, and
clothes

# LAYER 3

**Conventional**

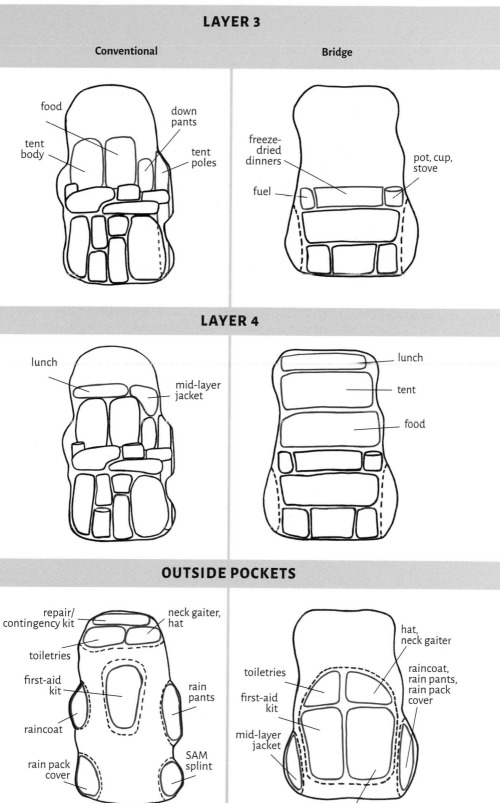

food

down pants

tent body

tent poles

**Bridge**

freeze-dried dinners

pot, cup, stove

fuel

# LAYER 4

lunch

mid-layer jacket

lunch

tent

food

# OUTSIDE POCKETS

repair/contingency kit

neck gaiter, hat

toiletries

first-aid kit

rain pants

raincoat

rain pack cover

SAM splint

hat, neck gaiter

toiletries

raincoat, rain pants, rain pack cover

first-aid kit

mid-layer jacket

repair/contingency kit

*The eye of danger and the face of fear are what really pull off a person's mask.*

—CRISS JAMI

## Assessing and Managing Risk

THERE IS SOME risk of danger inherent in all outdoor activities, but how can one judge the severity of unexpected challenges ahead of time? What criteria should we use to ensure our own—and our team's—safety?

The most important tool is a cool head. Thinking clearly and using common sense will go a long way toward sound decision-making. Understanding some basic risk-planning methods allows us to use those decisions wisely.

When I lead Grand Canyon treks, canyoneering trips, 14er trips, simple backpacks, or climbing trips, I go through a number of safety-related steps that are pretty automatic now for me, but can be explicitly defined. Below are the steps I take. These can be extrapolated to fit the planning for just about any kind of backcountry adventure:

1.  First and foremost, know the itinerary and the terrain that is involved. Study it, understand it, and get to know its dangers.

2.  Once this is understood, plan specific safety measures around the known risks expected in this trek. Ask yourself: Is any special equipment needed (for example, ropes or climbing gear, snowshoes, special clothing) to support these safety measures?

3.  Look at the trek from the contingency perspective. What are the unexpected dangers, risks, bizarre events that could happen? How can these be planned for, avoided, handled if they happen? How do these change the itinerary design? Do you need to take any additional gear to ensure the safety of the group in case of such events?

4.  What are the strengths and weaknesses of each person going on the trek? Who is the strongest, and who is the weakest? Who can be counted on for what in an emergency? Which ones are the dark horses who might save the day?

5. Taking all of the above into account, make final decisions on what kind of first-aid gear is needed on this trip and what kind of contingency gear should accompany the group.

6. What is the plan if the contingency plan doesn't work or cannot be implemented?

Now let's consider these steps through a couple of examples, so you can see why they matter and how to make this practical and appropriate for your own trips. These were real trips, but the planning is written in present tense to show how you might think through your own trip. A review of the events follows each example.

## EXAMPLE ONE

1. **THE ITINERARY FOR TRIP A:** a multiday backpack in the Grand Canyon that includes a one-day descent down a steep trail to a base camp, followed by several days of hiking local intra-canyon mesas in the area, and then a one-day ascent out of the canyon. We plan two driving days at the front and back, with five days of backpacking: two on either end for getting to and from camp, three for local exploration and fun.

   What are the dangers? This trail is steep, and people are carrying full packs. Normal considerations for steep hiking apply, namely, possible falls or trips and possible rock fall. The middle portion of the hike down to camp is a difficult trail with a cliff on one side; so another danger is that people could fall off the cliff. Once in camp, the dangers are those related to day hiking, climbing local peaks, and so on. In the canyon, this means steep hikes, slippery scree slopes, and again the dangers of falls, rock slides, and possible ankle injuries and such. We also must consider possible snake and scorpion bites as well as cactus and other pointy, injury-producing things in the canyon, along with normal considerations of sun exposure, dehydration, and so forth that usually accompany desert conditions. There are no major storms expected for this time, so weather is not a dangerous issue to be considered.

2. **SAFETY MEASURES FOR THESE RISKS:** Everyone should have trekking poles to assist during the steep descent and ascent with full packs. Everyone should have substantial footgear to support their descents and ascents on this rugged terrain, both in and out of camp.

A short piece of rope should be taken to be available as a hand-line in case the traverse near the cliff seems too dangerous to cross without it (because people are carrying full packs and might be frightened from the exposure due to the cliff). Two or more members of the party should be competent to set the hand-line properly to ensure safe use. Everyone will use 3-liter hydration systems with plenty of electrolyte-replacement foods included in their snacks. Everyone will have a sun hat, sunscreen, sunglasses, and so on.

3. **UNEXPECTED DANGERS:** What could happen? Well, anything! But the most bizarre thing we can think of might be a rockslide that might cut off part of the group from the rest, stranding some on one side of the slide and some on the other. Another possibility would be a heart attack, or someone buried in the rockslide. The only extra equipment might be another rope, possibly longer, and perhaps hand-held two-way radios for communication across the slide.

4. **STRENGTHS AND WEAKNESSES OF PARTICIPANTS:** This group is composed of 11 people, most strong hikers. One is older (in his 70s), and several others are veteran canyon backpackers. Most could be helpful in an emergency. Two have extensive first-aid training. The others have basic skills. Three people in particular are very strong and fast, so they could be counted on to help others.

5. **EXTRA GEAR NEEDED:** It is decided to take four radios and two 30-foot, 8-millimeter ropes, all divided among the group, with those leading and those at the back of the group having two of the radios in case we get spread out while hiking. Everyone is to bring a small first-aid kit. One person is assigned to bring a larger first-aid kit along with a SAM splint. We agree to regroup every hour while hiking, otherwise each can hike at their desired gait, as long as no person hikes alone. The trip is a hike-in, hike-out itinerary, so the basic contingency plan is to simply cut the trip short and come out if there is an emergency.

6. **LAST-RESORT PLAN:** The basic approach for this is, of course, we do the best we can! In this case, the contingency for the contingency is to send the strong ones for help.

This was good planning. Here's what actually happened:

On this Grand Canyon trek, we chose a trail called Nankoweep. It's 11 miles from car to camp, 3 miles of lovely gentle forest hiking, followed by a drop of 1,000 feet in 1 mile. This is followed by 4 miles of traverse on a trail that varies in width from 10 inches to 10 feet, filled with obstacles, with a cliff going up on the left and another cliff going down on the right. After this traverse, the trail drops another 3,000 vertical feet in 3 miles. So hikers must pay close attention for 8 miles in a row. This makes this trail, according to the National Park Service, the hardest trail in the canyon, perhaps because not everyone can focus carefully on every step for 8 miles continuously.

The group hiked the 3 miles of easy forest at the top just fine and descended the first 1,000 feet with no problem. During the traverse section, our group of 11 hikers spread out quite widely, and two things happened that were unexpected: One of the strong hikers had an old injury in his spine that he had failed to mention to the trip leader ahead of time. This created a bubble in the spinal cord, which turns him into a "space cadet" when he gets tired. So during the traverse, he spaced out, tripped, and fell, almost falling off the cliff. He managed to grab onto some tufts of grass on his way to the edge, then his hiking partners grabbed his backpack straps and pulled him back up and onto the trail, saving his life. (Only the three of them knew of this until we regrouped at the end of the day, because after a short rest he continued hiking with his partners carefully guiding him.)

The second event of the day was more serious in its impact. (And you thought falling off the cliff was bad . . . )

The oldest member of the party (whom I will call Sam, not his real name) was hiking much more slowly than the rest of us, so he ended up being the very last hiker in the group, hiking with one other person, a doctor, who patiently walked with him to ensure Sam was not hiking alone. This saved Sam's life. Halfway across the traverse, Sam began vomiting and collapsed in fatigue. When he began vomiting, the doctor examined him and concluded it was probably heat exhaustion because Sam did not complain of any other pain. He called on the radio communicating the situation. I was hiking with one other person about half a mile in front of these two, and as leader, I decided it was best for the rest of the group, now several miles ahead of Sam, to go on down to the creek for water and to set up camp. Furthermore, I decided we would hike to the end of the traverse to see how the situation evolved. The two of us hiked back to where Sam and the doctor were resting. We divided Sam's gear among the doctor and me so Sam had a very light pack, then continued hiking. Within half an hour, it became obvious that Sam could not make it to camp. We decided to bivouac on Tilted Mesa, the only flat area at the end of the traverse, just before the last 3 miles that drop 3,000 feet to camp. I radioed ahead for the group members who were not past that point to leave us what water they could spare, and to continue on down to the creek. I also instructed the group to camp without us and make do with the equipment they had, because we had divided up the group gear among all of us and a significant portion of that was among the four of us who would not be down at camp.

Three of us hiked with Sam to the end of the traverse and set up a dry (meaning we had no water source), makeshift camp there, giving what water we found left for us to Sam. We ate trail snacks and contingency food for dinner and breakfast. Tenting was interesting also, because my tent partner was down below with half of the tent while I was above with only the fly and stakes. It was good that we decided to divide it that way: He could actually set up the tent and sleep in it, while I used the fly as a ground cloth to sleep under the stars. Others had similar arrangements. Very lucky that it did not rain that night. In the morning we arranged via radio for two hikers to come meet us with water to rehydrate us, along with empty packs so they could take Sam's gear to camp. By the time they arrived, Sam was feeling better but not great. We slowly walked him down to camp and arranged for him to rest. At this point it was obvious that we had a serious situation. I called for a group meeting to discuss options. During the discussion it became clear that the situation was even worse than it appeared on the surface. As we spoke with each member of the group, almost everyone had some sort of injury causing them pain. Some were known knee injuries that were now causing pain, others were old ankle injuries resurfacing. All but 3 of the 11 people on the trek were impaired in some way! As leader I needed the contingency for the contingency for the contingency!

I suggested we change our itinerary completely to abandon our plans and simply ensure the safety of all involved. We changed the trip to have one layover rest day followed by a two-day ascent back to the cars. In order to do the ascent, we needed to have water for our dry camp on Tilted Mesa. Three brave and strong souls (the only three still uninjured) emptied their packs of gear, filled them with containers full of water, and hiked up to the mesa to leave a water cache, returning to camp to pick up their gear for the hike out. We divided up Sam's gear among us all, hiking slowly to prevent further injuries as best we could. We took two full days to come out, and we all lived to tell about it. In this way everyone was able to hike out, including Sam, who, when he got home, found out he had a hernia!

## Lessons Learned

Several factors prevented this trip from becoming tragic:

- ⚙ The radios were central to the success of the trip. Without them it would have been difficult to communicate what was happening and to arrange for water and the means to carry Sam's gear the next day.

- ⚙ Individuals were willing to give up personal goals for the safety of the group, and everyone was willing to change plans to ensure we all got home safely. This made the change of itinerary work.

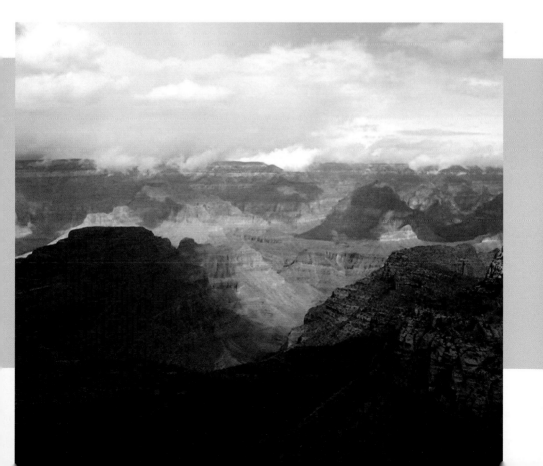

◉    Volunteers who were willing to hike an extra 6 miles and 6,000 vertical feet with heavy packs helped ensure our safe exit, and allowed us to survive this in relative luxury.

◉    It was critical to have one person in charge willing to discuss options with the group and make decisions. These decisions were made calmly rather than in a panic. Everyone accepted those decisions.

◉    No ropes were needed, but one section of trail was so narrow that some members of the group asked me to carry their packs over that part so they could cross more safely. There were no rockslides or heart attacks, but the contingency considerations that caused us to bring radios for those conditions played a large role in what did happen.

## EXAMPLE TWO

1.  **The itinerary for Trip B:** a Grand Canyon trip that is planned as a simple backpacking trip for four people to the Hermit Creek area, with a couple of nights at Monument Creek. This is a straightforward hike-in, set-up-camp, layover-day, hike-out kind of trip. Risks for this trip are just those of hiking on a steep backcountry trail, namely, possible falls, knee or ankle injuries, and so on, the normal kind of thing we expect to handle on a steep hike with a pack. No cliff exposure or unusual circumstances expected.

2.  **Unexpected dangers:** Because it's a hike with packs on a good but steep trail, safety measures include a first-aid kit for each participant. One of us will bring a SAM splint and larger kit, and everyone will have good footgear, trekking poles, and be in good physical shape. No weather systems are expected, so no unusual weather protection is deemed necessary.

3.  **Contingency plans:** These are contained in the normal safety measures, so the only contingencies are possible alternative itineraries.

4.  **Strengths and weaknesses of participants:** This group is composed of a close friend, his girlfriend, and his son (whom I will call John, not his real name), who is in his 20s and very strong. All except

the girlfriend are experienced backpackers who also have experience with first aid and rock climbing.

5. **Extra gear needed:** Because this is such a well-known trail, no additional contingency equipment is deemed necessary.

6. **Last-resort plan:** A bit of extra food is included in case of an unexpected delay.

Here is what happened on this trip:

The backpack went perfectly according to plan until we were hiking out on the last day. About halfway up the Hermit Creek Trail, we came around a bend to find a woman lying in the trail. Her friends were sitting nearby in the shade of a large boulder, while the woman just rested in the middle of the trail. We learned she had hurt her ankle and was in great pain. The friends had no clue what to do. So we treated this woman for shock, taped her ankle (assuming it was badly sprained), put it back into her boot and installed the SAM splint around the boot to hold the ankle in place. We gave her food and water, got her back to a reasonably healthy state, and then took all of the gear from John's pack and distributed it among our packs, leaving John's pack empty. We then put the woman's pack into John's pack (it fit perfectly), so John could carry it out. We gave the woman a daypack to carry food and water for the trip out, and we made arrangements where to leave her gear at the top. Since she had trekking poles to use as crutches, we expected her to limp slowly to the top with her friends beside her. We then hiked out, carrying her gear.

At the top we left her pack at the arranged place, with a note as to who we were and how to contact us, and proceeded on our way to Flagstaff and home. After some months of not hearing a word, I got a phone call out of the blue. The woman had misplaced our sheet of paper and just found it, some 10 months after our trip. She told me this story: After we left her, she tried to limp up the trail but found it too painful. Incredibly, her friends had gone on ahead leaving her to hike alone. She finally began crawling (!) up the trail, and after some time, to her amazement, a hiker came along who dumped his pack, put her on his back and carried her to the top. She eventually got to the Flagstaff hospital where they found she had broken her ankle in three places. After surgery and months of recovery she was able to walk normally again. The doctor at the hospital was impressed with the stabilization of her ankle, and she thanked us for our help and apologized for the delay in contacting us.

## Lessons Learned

This was one of three times I have had to use a SAM splint in the wild to treat a serious ankle injury in the past 20 years. Two of the three instances were broken ankles, the third a bad sprain. At the time it seemed that knowing how to handle the situation from a first-aid perspective made it fairly simple. However, we made some false assumptions that turned out to complicate the patient's situation to the extent that her life became endangered:

⚙    We assumed that the group dynamic in her group was similar to those we practice, that is, that members of the group care about the safety and health of other members of the group.

⚙    We assumed she could walk on her ankle.

⚙    Although she had food and water in her day pack, she was not in a mental state to use these things wisely, as she was experiencing extreme pain and fatigue.

Although we planned for and used contingency first-aid supplies and skill, we did not plan for or understand the social situation. In hindsight we should have insisted that she hike with us, or at least we should have discussed the seriousness of the situation with her hiking group, the other three women who abandoned her.

What do these two examples teach about risk management? Here are some thoughts:

⚙    Risk-management strategy, contingency planning, and being as prepared as you can be are only the starting points. We have no control over what will present itself to us in the middle of a trek. We have knowledge, preparations, and our gear. We also have our ability to observe what is happening around us. These are our tools. This is where we begin.

⚙    When the event unfolds, we must combine our ability to observe with what we know to try to make sense of what is presented to us. From that, we can see what our choices are. Then we make the best choice based on the conditions in which we find ourselves, the input from trusted friends, the equipment we have with us, and the immediacy of the situation.

- Once in it, we must be flexible, creative, and engaged with the situation while at the same time remaining aloof from it enough to not be blinded by its overwhelming nature. Remaining calm and making clear and definitive decisions are helpful, even if those decisions are the wrong ones.

- Following up after an event is prudent and could save a life. In some situations this is not necessary (as in the first example, where all of the parties involved were together); in others, it may seem unnecessary but is paramount (as in example B, where the victim was separated from the caregivers). Debriefing discussions among participants also can provide great learning opportunities.

- In practice, risk assessment and management are actually a combination of the following:

  - learning, planning, and preparation prior to the trip
  - personal experience and knowledge from life and previous trips
  - the circumstances of the event
  - the terrain and the weather conditions in which the event occurs
  - the equipment involved
  - the people involved
  - the social situation
  - the decision possibilities and choices presented
  - who is making decisions
  - whether the decision maker is able to be aware of what is happening around him or her
  - who is available to help the decision maker in discussing options
  - the decisions made and their consequences
  - how well the people involved are able to deal with the situation as presented, the decisions made, and the outcome

In all contingency situations, communication is a key player. No matter what your risk-management technique, or what unfolds, clear communication among all involved will help.

Furthermore, our strategy and ability to manage risks can be impacted by our choice of gear, conventional or ultralight. In some cases, conventional backpacks are better prepared for contingency than ultralight, simply because there is often

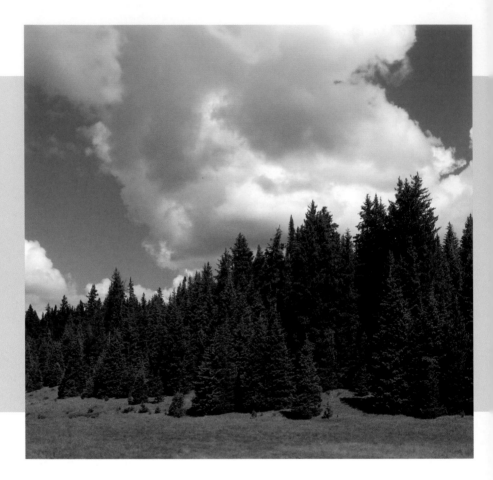

more gear to use in an emergency, and there is stronger gear for unconventional use (like using a backpack as a litter or, as in Example Two, John's using his conventional pack to carry someone else's full pack). However, with an ultralight load, sometimes the difficulty of the situation is lessened. For example, the injured backpacker in example A, who could no longer carry his pack, required others to carry his gear. If his pack had been ultralight, it would not have weighed the conventional 40–50 pounds, but rather perhaps 20–25 pounds; thus, dividing that weight among other members of the group would have been much easier.

In addition, the ultralight principle of being able to use gear for multiple purposes shines in the arena of risk contingency planning. Knowing first-aid and repair techniques that employ backpacking gear as tools is essential, especially when ultralight or bridge gear is used. Some simple examples of this might be the following: using a shirt to create a sling for a broken arm, applying a 1-inch nylon strap to hold a bandage in place, using an ultralight or bridge backpack as a splint or as part of the bandage for an injured leg, and, of course, using tent poles or trekking poles as splints, and so on. Similarly, being creative with gear to help keep someone warm and dry can save a trip or even a life. For more on this topic, see the contingency-planning discussions in previous chapters for both three-season treks (page 76) and winter adventures (page 114). And remember that under some conditions we might have to sacrifice gear or leave some gear behind to save a life or a limb—a decision that must be made on the spot.

 ## Quick Tips

 Risk assessment is a task not only for the trip leader but also for everyone who ventures into the wilderness.

✓ Combining common sense with being well prepared allows us to participate in things that push our limits. Knowing how to safely navigate during such times reduces fear and helps us more calmly deal with events.

✓ Risk assessment is not just about knowing how to best decide what to do—it is also about knowing how to effectively use whatever gear we have on hand in unusual circumstances.

✓ With larger groups where hikers tend to spread out on the trail, you can better ensure safety when the terrain is rough by asking each hiker to keep an eye on the person behind them. As long as they can see the person behind them, they can continue hiking. If they cannot, they should stop to wait for that person. If he/she doesn't come, perhaps something is wrong. This procedure can help to quickly assess problems and get help when needed. It also helps slower or beginner hikers to feel safer and more supported in difficult hiking conditions.

> *S*low down and enjoy life. It's not only the scenery you miss by going too fast —you also miss the sense of where you are going and why.
>
> —EDDIE CANTOR

## Effective Trip Planning

THE CHOICE OF CONVENTIONAL or ultralight gear feeds into the overall planning process for backcountry trekking. A well-planned trek is usually a much more fun trip with minimized chances for problems. Here are the guidelines I teach to help people plan better treks. (Steps Two and Three can be interchanged if you really want to visit a specific place. You can select the destination, and then decide how difficult you want your trek to be in that general location. These two steps together dictate a specific set of possible choices from which you create itineraries, as in Step Four.)

1. Decide with whom you want to share this trek.

2. Decide the desired difficulty of the trip, perhaps from combinations of the following list of choices:

   - backpacking
   - beginner conditions
   - canyoneering
   - desert conditions
   - difficult terrain or advanced conditions
   - high altitude
   - rock climbing
   - simple hiking
   - skiing or snowshoeing
   - winter conditions

3. Decide the locations available based on Step Two above, and choose two or three of those that seem appropriate.

4. Write out possible itineraries for these choices.

5. Choose first- and second-choice itineraries that are the best suited for the people involved.

6. Decide the best time of year for these two trek itineraries. Pick specific dates for the trek you are planning.

7. Invite the list of potential participants.

8. Pick one itinerary and adjust dates and plans based on who can go, weather predictions, gear availability, vehicle availability, and so on. Finalize your list of participants and dates based on the new plans.

9. Lay out exact details of the trip logistics.

10. Contact local authorities to find out the latest information for the trek area—trail, forest, or road closures; avalanche, fire, flash flood, storm warnings, or wind; river, road, slope, snowpack, and trail conditions; expected weather conditions and locations of water sources; and expected hiking conditions and general safety information.

11. Have a trip-planning meeting. I usually have a potluck dinner meeting to go over every detail of the trip. It is best if all participants can attend. This meeting should cover:

    a. specifics of the trip itinerary

    b. pre- and post-trek hotels or campsites

    c. travel logistics

    d. hiking logistics

    e. meals and cooking

    f. water availability

    g. group gear that is shared (some examples listed below, but don't be limited to these):
       - dining fly
       - first-aid kit(s)
       - shelters
       - specialty gear (like climbing ropes)
       - stoves, pots, and fuel
       - water purification and storage

       h.    personal gear

       i.    tenting arrangements

       j.    finances

       k.    contingency plans

       l.    training events

12.   Address any participant concerns.

13.   Execute your plan. Make it fun.

14.   Take notes on what worked and what didn't. Learn from your mistakes.

A note about trip-planning contingencies: On one of our early trips to the Grand Canyon, we had four vehicles traveling some 500 miles to get to the South Rim, where we were to camp. I rode with my wife and daughter, who, on this trip, were going to stay in a hotel on the Rim and day hike while the rest of us were backpacking. My friend Rick drove his new truck, while other

 ## *Quick Tips*

 It is important to remember that you, the trip leader, do not need to be responsible for everything. You are responsible for organizing the trek and getting it started. Delegation involves trip participants so they own the trip, too.

 I find it extremely useful to have one participant delegated to be the trip navigator. This person is in charge of the map and compass and perhaps a GPS, and ensures that the group does not get lost. The leader is still responsible for making sure individual members don't wander off.

✓ Having a pre-trip potluck dinner meeting to plan everything helps ensure that everyone is informed and that all equipment and planning are understood. It also helps the group bond prior to the trip. Having a celebratory dinner after the trek to share "war stories" and pictures from the trip rounds out the fun.

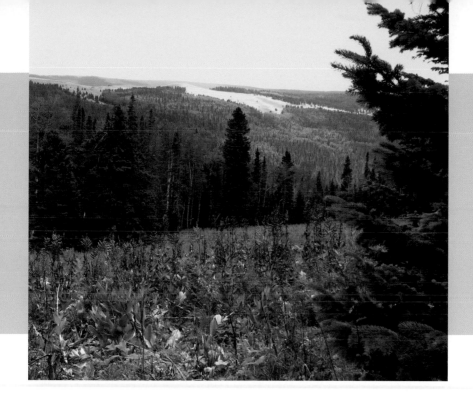

vehicles carried other participants. When my car arrived in a raging snowstorm at Mather Campground, my wife dropped me off to meet the group, while she and my daughter went to check into their hotel. We expected Rick and the others to show up any minute. There was one other person at the campsite when I arrived, so we proceeded to set up a tarp under which we could huddle while we awaited our jackets, tents, and other gear that were in the back of Rick's truck. In the meantime, Rick's new truck had some trouble, so they pulled into a gas station to have it checked. The mechanic put the truck up on the garage lift to work on it and, due to the chilly temperatures, closed the garage door. That's when the power went out. They then discovered a rather important thing. There was no manual way to open the garage door. It was a new design and was implemented improperly. So Rick spent some three hours in that garage waiting for the power to come back on! In the meantime, we were huddled under a tarp watching the now-8-inch-deep snow get deeper. None of us had phones or radios. All we could do was wait. Eventually our gear showed up and the trip continued uneventfully. However, we learned that we needed a way to communicate between vehicles in transit, and we learned not to separate ourselves from our gear.

*Life is a perpetual joy of exploring and living in a continuous state of wonder and awe.*

—PETER CAJANDER

## Living with Your Choices and Evolving with the Times

FOCUS ON THE JOY that comes from being in the backcountry, and let your gear be the support mechanism helping to create that joy. Using the principles outlined in this book, try adjusting your base weight down a number of pounds. Experiment with lighter-weight gear while continuing to evolve skills and abilities as backpackers. Your abilities to use gear in more effective ways will increase and grow, just as the technology to create lighter gear continues to create more choices.

Over time you may have to revisit this process as newer gear becomes available. That's inherent in using gear that is continually improving. Enjoy the process, and never forget what a gift the wilderness is to us.

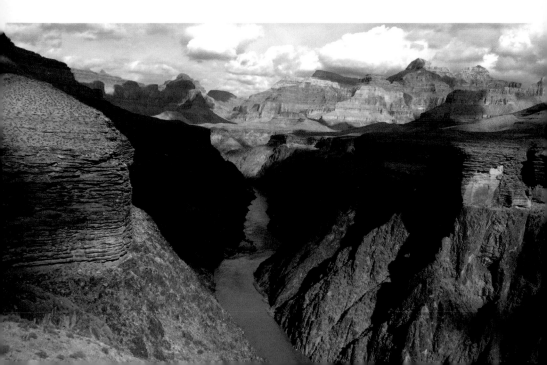

# Resources

## Web-Based Resources

Here are a few good websites focused on ultralight backpacking. (There are many more; I haven't listed many here, because too soon they all will be obsolete.)

**adventurealan.com**

**andrewskurka.com**

**backpacking.net**

**backpackinglight.com**

**hikelight.com**

**ultralightbackpacker.com**

These websites offer good general backpacking advice, relevant articles, and gear comparisons:

**backpacker.com**

**cleverhiker.com**

**rei.com/expertadvice/camping**

**sectionhiker.com**

# Books Proven to be Good Backpacking Resources

*Allen & Mike's Really Cool Backpackin' Book,* by Allen O'Bannon and Mike Clelland

*AMC Guide to Outdoor Leadership,* by Alex Kosseff

*Backcountry Nutrition,* by Mary Howley Ryan
(a National Outdoor Leadership School [NOLS] book)

*Hiking and Backpacking,* by Victoria Logue

*Hiking and Backpacking: A Complete Illustrated Guide,* by Buck Tilton and
Stephen Gorman

*The Joy of Backpacking,* by Brian Belfort

*Lighten Up! A Complete Handbook for Light and Ultralight Backpacking,*
by Don Ladigin

*Lightweight Backpacking and Camping,* by Ryan Jordan

*Mountaineering: The Freedom of the Hills,* by The Mountaineers (a Mountaineers book)

*The National Outdoor Leadership School's Wilderness Guide,* by Mark Harvey
(an NOLS book)

*NOLS Cookery,* by Claudia Pearson (an NOLS book)

*The Outward Bound Backpacker's Handbook,* by Glen Randall

*The Outward Bound Wilderness First-Aid Handbook,* by Jeffrey Isaac

*The Ultralight Backpacker,* by Ryel Kestenbaum

*Ultralight Backpackin' Tips,* by Mike Clelland

*Wilderness Basics,* Fourth Edition, San Diego Sierra Club (a Mountaineers book)

*Wilderness First Aid,* by Tod Schimelpfenig, Linda Lindsey, and Joan Safford
(an NOLS book)

*Wilderness Mountaineering,* by Phil Powers (an NOLS book)

*Winter Camping,* by John Gookin and Buck Tilton (an NOLS book)

# Image Credits

| PAGE | DESCRIPTION (+ caption where applicable) | ARTIST | YEAR CREATED |
|---|---|---|---|
| v | Chama River Valley | Richard Moeller | 2013 |
| ix | East side of Santa Fe Baldy Peak from Pecos Baldy Trail | Richard Moeller | 2008 |
| x | Cumbres Pass Area | Richard Moeller | 2008 |
| 6 | Rick's dog, Bruce (*Bruce knows comfort. Do you?*) | Richard A. Light | 2014 |
| 9 | Santa Fe National Forest | Richard Moeller | 2008 |
| 10 | Santa Fe National Forest | Richard Moeller | 2008 |
| 14 | Santa Fe Baldy Peak from Raven's Ridge Trail | Richard Moeller | 2007 |
| 17 | Lake Peak from Puerto Nambe (*Why am I here?*) | Richard Moeller | 2007 |
| 22 | Vase/faces optical illusion (*What do you see?*) | Public domain | Unknown |
| 22 | Young/old optical illusion (*What do you see?*) | Public Domain | Unknown |
| 29 | Ash and Ian hiking the Bear Lake Trail | Richard Moeller | 2009 |
| 35 | Bear Lake | Richard Moeller | 2009 |
| 36 | Scale weighing gear (*A kitchen scale works well for weighing gear.*) | Thea Rose Light | 2014 |
| 38 | Pecos Baldy Lake | Richard A. Light | 2014 |
| 40 | Full backpacks (*My Conventional Pack, My Bridge Pack*) | Thea Rose Light | 2014 |
| 44 | Ultralight packs (*What features do you need in your ultralight pack?*) Courtesy of GoLite, Gossamer Gear, Granite Gear, Mountain Laurel Designs, Six Moons Designs, ULA Equipment, and Zpacks | | Unknown |
| 45 | Trekking poles (*Twist-Style vs. Cam-Style Trekking Poles*) | Thea Rose Light | 2014 |
| 48 | Clothing layers | Thea Rose Light | 2014 |
| 50 | Rain-pant comparison (*Conventional rain pants are heavier than Cuben Fiber rain pants.*) | Thea Rose Light | 2014 |
| 55 | Shoes and boots comparison (*For each specific trip, pick the right kind of foot gear.*) | Thea Rose Light | 2014 |
| 59 | Tents and shelters (*What kind of shelter meets your needs?*) Courtesy of Big Agnes, Cascade Designs, GoLite, Nova Equipment, Six Moons Designs, Tarptent, Terra, and Zpacks | | Unknown |
| 60 | Hubba and Hexamid tent comparison (*Conventional MSR Hubba or the ultralight Zpacks Hexamid Solo Plus?*) | Thea Rose Light | 2014 |
| 63 | EN testing tag (*European Norm Testing Tag for Sleeping Bags*) | Thea Rose Light | 2014 |
| 65 | Sleeping pads (*Pad design affects weight, cushion, and insulation.*) | Thea Rose Light | 2014 |

*(Continued on next page)*

| PAGE | DESCRIPTION (+ caption where applicable) | ARTIST | YEAR CREATED |
|---|---|---|---|
| 68 | View from Monument Creek, Grand Canyon | Richard A. Light | 2014 |
| 70, 71 | First-aid kit and SAM splint (First-Aid Kit) | Thea Rose Light | 2014 |
| 72 | Knife, multitool, razor blade (How much of a cutting tool do you need?) | Thea Rose Light | 2014 |
| 80 | Stoves / Courtesy of Cascade Designs, Esbit, Soto, and public domain | | Unknown |
| 88 | Water filters and drops | Thea Rose Light | 2014 |
| 89 | Water containers and bladders | Thea Rose Light | 2014 |
| 92 | Specialty gear | Thea Rose Light | 2014 |
| 94 | Pecos Wilderness | Richard Moeller | 2008 |
| 96 | Lake Peak in winter from Raven's Ridge Trail | Richard Moeller | 2008 |
| 99 | Insulated pants, hiking pants (Your metabolism dictates what layers will work best.) | Thea Rose Light | 2014 |
| 100 | Winter boots, snowshoes, skis | Thea Rose Light | 2014 |
| 104 | Winter stove platform | Richard A. Light | 2013 |
| 106 | Winter tent with author in doorway (Donning boots at the door of a four-season tent. Note the snow saw and shovel used to create a place to sit.) | Ash Campbell | 2010 |
| 107 | Igloo with gear locker and Ash (My friend Ash enjoying the porch of a newly completed igloo. Note the gear storage shed behind him, and the door to the interior on the right.) | Cameron Gay | 2011 |
| 108 | Icebox igloo off Nambe Lake Trail | Richard Moeller | 2007 |
| 108 | Snow shelter in drift atop Raven's Ridge | Tim Burns | 2010 |
| 108 | Snow house with vigas at Puerto Nambe | Ash Campbell | 2010 |
| 110 | Sleeping-pad comparison for winter | Thea Rose Light | 2014 |
| 111 | Big Tesuque Creek in winter | Richard Moeller | 2005 |
| 113 | Snowshoes and skis | Thea Rose Light | 2014 |
| 115 | Personal locator beacons Courtesy of ACR Electronics, Spot LLC, and DeLorme | | 2014 |
| 116 | Hoar frost in early morning | Richard Moeller | 2008 |
| 118 | Santa Fe National Forest | Richard Moeller | 2008 |
| 123 | Reflection in pond | Richard Moeller | 2008 |
| 125 | Figure 1: How to Balance Gear Inside the Pack | Morgan Light | 2014 |
| 127 | Figure 2: Pack-Strap Labels | Morgan Light | 2014 |
| 128,129 | Diagram of layers in a pack | Morgan Light | 2014 |
| 135 | View of Grand Canyon | Richard A. Light | 2011 |
| 140 | Pecos Wilderness | Richard Moeller | 2008 |
| 145 | Pecos Wilderness | Richard A. Light | 2014 |
| 146 | Colorado River, Grand Canyon | Richard A. Light | 2014 |

# Index

# About the Author

RICHARD A. LIGHT is an instructor of backpacking, rock climbing, and other outdoor skills. He has been backpacking, climbing, hiking, skiing, and generally active in the outdoors for more than 50 years. He especially loves telemark skiing, rock climb-

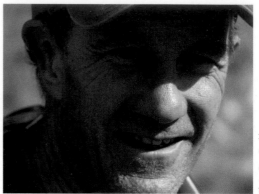

Photo: Dave Scudder

ing, backpacking, canyoneering, snowshoeing, building igloos, and reveling in the beauty and majesty of nature. Rick taught skiing as an RMSIA/PSIA fully certified alpine instructor in the late 1960s and early 1970s. He has been designing and leading multiday backpacks in remote areas of the Grand Canyon since 1993. He loves playing in the high country above timberline, canyoneering through slot canyons, exploring backcountry with no trails, teaching and helping others, and, especially, just being in the silence and wonder of wilderness. He lives in Santa Fe, New Mexico.